The Vitamine Manual

by Walter H. Eddy

CONTENTS

The presentation of essential data concerning vitamines to succeeding groups of students has become increasingly difficult with the development of research in this field. The literature itself has assumed a bulk that precludes sending the student to original sources except in those instances when they are themselves to become investigators. The demand on the part of the layman for concise information about the new food factors is increasing and worthy of attention. For all of these reasons it has seemed worth while to collate the existing data and put it in a form which would be available for both student and layman. Such is the purpose of this little book.

It has been called a manual since the arrangement aims to provide the student with working material and suggestions for investigation as well as information. The bibliography, the data in the chapter on vitamine testing, the tables and the subdivision of subject matter have all been arranged to aid the laboratory workers and it is the hope that this plan may make the manual of especial value to the student investigator. The management also separates the details necessary to laboratory investigation from the more purely historical aspects of the subject which we believe will be appreciated by the lay reader as well as the student.

No apologies are made for data which on publication shall be found obsolete. The whole subject is in too active a state of investigation to permit of more than a record of events and their apparent bearing. Whenever there is controversy the aim has been to cite opposing views and indicate their apparent value but with full realization that this value may be profoundly altered by new data.

Since the type of the present manual was set, Drummond of England has suggested that we drop the terminal "e" in Vitamine, since the ending "ine" has a chemical significance which is to date not justified as a termination for the name of the unidentified dietary factors. This suggestion has been generally adopted by research workers and the spelling now in use is Vitamin A, B, or C. It has hardly seemed worth while to derange the entire set up of the present text to make this correction and we have retained the form in use at the time the manuscript was first set up. The suggestion of Drummond, however, is sound and will undoubtedly be generally adopted by the research workers in the subject.

Attempt has been made to cover all the important contributions up to April, 1921. Opportunity has permitted the inclusion of certain data of still later date and undoubtedly other important papers of earlier date will have been overlooked.

It is a pleasure to acknowledge the assistance received in the preparation of the manuscript from Dr. H. C. Sherman, Dr. Mary S. Rose and Dr. Victor La Mer. Their suggestions have been most valuable and greatly appreciated.

WALTER H. EDDY.

Department of Physiological Chemistry, Teachers College, Columbia University, New York City, April, 1921

CHAPTER I

HOW VITAMINES WERE DISCOVERED

In 1911 Casimir Funk coined the name Vitamine to describe the substance which he believed curative of an oriental disease known as beri-beri. This disease is common in Japan, the Philippines and other lands where the diet consists mainly of rice, and while the disease itself was well known its cause and cure had baffled the medical men for many years. Today in magazines, newspapers and street car advertisements people are urged to use this or that food or medicament on the plea of its vitamine content. In less than ten years the study of vitamines has increased to such an extent that it is difficult to find a chemical journal of any month of issue that does not contain one or more articles bearing on the subject. Such a rapid rise to public notice suggests an importance that justifies investigation by the laity as well as the chemist and in the pages that follow has been outlined in simple language the biography of this newest and lustiest of the chemist's children.

Dr. Funk christened one individual but the family has grown since 1911 to three members which for lack of better names are now called vitamines "A," "B," and "C." There are now rumors of another arrival and none dare predict the limits of the family. Had these new substances been limited to their relation to an obscure oriental disease they would have of course commanded the medical attention but it is doubtful whether the general public would have found it worth while to concern themselves. It is because on better acquaintance they have compelled us to reform our ideas on nutrition of both adults and babies and pick out our foods from a new angle, that we accord them the attention they demand and deserve. Granting then, their claim upon our attention, let us review our present knowledge and try to see with just what we are dealing. This will be more easily accomplished if we consider the vitamines first from the historical side and reserve our attention to details of behavior until later.

A limited diet of polished rice and fish is a staple among the peoples of the Orient. When the United States Government took over the Philippine Islands in 1898 it sent there a small group of scientists to establish laboratories and become acquainted with the peculiarities of the people and their troubles. One of the first matters that engaged their attention was the condition of the prisons which were most unsanitary and whose inhabitants were poorly fed and treated. Reforms were put into operation at once and the sanitary measures soon changed these prisons to places not quite so abhorrent to the eye. In trying to improve the diets of the prisoners little change was made in their composition because of the native habits but the reformers saw to it that the rice fed should be clean and white. In spite of these measures the first year saw a remarkable increase in the disease of beri-beri, and the little group of laboratory scientists had at once before them the problem of checking a development that bid fair to become an epidemic. In fact, the logical discoverers of what we now know as the antineuritic vitamine or vitamine "B" should have been this same group of laboratory workers for it was largely due to their work between the years 1900 and 1911 that the ground was prepared for Funk's harvest.

The relation of rice to this disease was more than a suspicion even in 1898. In 1897 a Dutch chemist, Eijkman, had succeeded in producing in fowls a similar set of symptoms by feeding them with polished rice alone. This set of symptoms he called polyneuritis and this term is now commonly used to signify a beri-beri in experimental animals. Eijkman found that two or three weeks feeding sufficed to produce these symptoms and it was he who first showed that the addition of the rice polishings to the diet was sufficient to relieve the symptoms. Eijkman first thought that the cortical material contained something necessary to neutralize the effects of a diet rich in starch. Later however, he changed his view and in 1906 his position was practically the view of today. In that same year (1906) F. Gowland Hopkins in England had come to the conclusion that the growth of laboratory animals demanded something in foods that could not be accounted for among the ordinary nutrients. He gave to these hypothetical substances the name "accessory food factors." To Hopkins and to Eijkman may therefore be justly attributed the credit of calling the world's attention to the unknown substances which Funk was to christen a little later with the name vitamines. Other workers, of course, knew of these experiments of Eijkman and Hopkins and in 1907 two of them, Fraser and Stanton, reported that by extracting rice polishings with alcohol they had secured a product which if added to the diet of a sufferer from beri-beri seemed to produce curative effects. It is obvious that logic would have decreed that some of these workers should be the ones to identify and name the curative material. But history is not bound by the rules of logic and it was so in this case. Another student had been attracted to the problem and was working at the time in Germany where he also became acquainted with Eijkman's results and began the investigation of rice polishings on experimental lines. This student was Casimir Funk and a little later he carried his studies to England where he developed the results that made him the first to announce the discovery of the unknown factor which he christened vitamine. Funk's studies combined a careful chemical fractioning of the extracts of rice polishings with tests for their antineuritic power upon polyneuritic birds, after the manner taught by Eijkman. By carrying out this fractioning and testing he obtained from a large volume of rice polishings a very small amount of a crystalline substance which proved to be curative to a high degree. A little later he demonstrated that this same substance was particularly abundant in brewers' yeast. From these two sources he obtained new extracts and carefully repeated his analytical fractionings. The result was the demonstration that they contained a substance which could be reduced to crystalline form and was therefore worthy of being considered a chemical substance. In 1911, before Fraser and Stanton or any other workers had been able to show to what their curative extracts were due, Funk produced his product, demonstrated its properties and claimed his right to naming the same. At that he barely escaped priority from still another source. The chemists in Japan were naturally interested in this problem and possessed an able worker by the name of Suzuki. Suzuki and his co-workers Odake and Shimamura were engaged in the same fractioning processes with polishings and entirely independently of Funk or other workers they too succeeded in isolating a curative substance and published their discovery the same year as Funk, 1911. Their methods were later shown to be identical up to a certain point. Suzuki called his product "Oryzanin." Funk's elementary analyses had shown the presence of nitrogen in this product and his method of extraction indicated that this nitrogen was present in basic form. For that reason he suggested that his product belonged to a class of substances which chemists call "amines." Since its absence meant death and its presence life what more natural than to call it the Life-amine or Vita-amine. This is the origin of Funk's nomenclature.

Both Funk's original crystals and Suzuki's oryzanin were later shown to be complexes of the curative substances combined with adulterants and we do not yet know just what a vitamine is or whether it is an amine at all but no one since 1911 has been able to get any nearer to the identification than Funk and while he has added much data to his earlier studies he has himself not yet given us the pure vitamine. For that reason it has been suggested by various people that the name vitamine should not be used since it has no sufficient evidence to support it. Hopkins of England had suggested the name "accessory food factors." E. V. McCollum holds that we should call them the "unidentified dietary factors" and added later to this phrase, the terms water-soluble "B" and fat-soluble "A" after the fat soluble form was discovered. Most chemists feel, however, that the purpose of nomenclature is brevity combined with ready recognition of what you are discussing and that it is unnecessary to change the name vitamine until we know exactly what the substances are. The result is that while still a mystery chemically they remain under the name of vitamine and the kinds are distinguished by the McCollum terms "fat-soluble" A, "water-soluble" B, and "C."

We see that beri-beri then was responsible for Funk's adding to our chemical entities a new member but it does not yet appear why this entity concerns our normal nutrition. To get this relation we must turn for a moment to the state of knowledge in 1911 in regard to foods and their evaluation and what was going on in this field of study at the time.

A great advance in measuring food value was the discovery of the isodynamic law. Translated into ordinary language this law states that when a person eats a given amount of a given kind of food, that food may liberate in the body practically the same amount of energy that it would produce if it were burned in oxygen outside of the body. The confirmation of this law permitted us to apply to the measurement of food the same method we had already learned to use in measuring coal. For convenience the physicists devised a heat measure unit for this purpose and naturally called it by a word that means heat, namely, "calorie." Using this unit and applying the isodynamic law it was merely necessary to determine two things; first, how many calories a man produces in any given kind of work, second how many calories a given weight of each kind of food will yield, and then give the man as many calories of food as he needs to meet his requirements when engaged in a given kind of labor. The measurement and tabulation of food values in terms of calories and the investigation of the calorie needs of men and women in various occupations has been one of the great contributions of the past twenty years of nutritional study and to the progress made we owe our power to produce proper rations for every type of worker. Army rations for example are built up of foods that will yield enough calories to supply the needs of a soldier and during the recent war extended studies conducted in training camps all over the United States have shown that when the soldier eats all he wants he will consume on the average about 3600 calories per day. In France the American soldier's ration was big enough to yield him 4200 calories per day if he ate his entire daily allowance.

But calories are not the only necessities. A pound of pure fat will yield all the calories a soldier needs in a day but his language and morals wouldn't stand the strain of such a diet. Neither would his health, for not only does his body demand fuel but also that it be of a special kind. While there are many kinds of foodstuffs, chemical analysis shows that they are mainly combinations of pure compounds of relatively few varieties. The chemists call these proteins, fats, carbohydrates, and salts. Meats, eggs, the curd of milk, etc., are the principal sources of protein. Sugars and starches are grouped together under the name of carbohydrate. By salts is meant mineral matters such as common salt, iron and phosphorus compounds, etc. In selecting foods it was found that the body required that the proportions of these four substances be kept within definite limits or there was trouble. We know now that a man can get along nicely if he eats 50 grams of protein per day and makes up the rest of his calories in carbohydrates and fats, provided that to this is added certain requirements in salts and water.

It is also obvious that the foods given must be digestible and palatable.

We had reached this status some time before 1911. But, a short time before this, there had arisen a controversy as to the relative value of different types of proteins. The animal- vs. vegetable-protein controversy was one of the side shows of this affair. This controversy had led to a careful study of the different kinds of proteins that are found in foodstuffs. Through a brilliant series of chemical investigations for whose description we haven't time or space here, chemists had shown that every protein was built up of a collection of acids which were different in structure and properties, that there were some seventeen of these in all and that any given protein might have present all seventeen or be lacking in one or more and that the proportions present varied for every type of protein. It was then obvious that proteins could not be considered as identities. More than that, it was the necessary task of the food expert to separate all proteins into their acids or building stones and not only show what was present and how much but determine the role each played in the body. To this task many set their faces and hands.

From the results there has accrued much progress in the evaluation of proteins but an unexpected development was the part played by these investigations in the story of the vitamines.

About 1909-1910 Professors Osborne and Mendel under a grant from the Carnegie Institution began a detailed investigation into the value of purified proteins from various sources. In their experiments they used the white rat as the experimental animal and proceeded to feed these animals a mixture consisting of a single purified protein supplemented with the proper proportions of fat carbohydrate, and mineral salts. Since the food furnished was composed of pure nutrients and always in excess of the appetite of the rat the necessary number of calories was also present. These researches were published as a bulletin (No. 156) by the Carnegie Institution in 1911, the same year that Funk announced his Vitamine discoveries. It was timely in this respect for one of Osborne and Mendel's discoveries was that no matter how efficient the mixture in all the requirements then known to the nutrition expert, the rats failed to grow unless there was added to the diet a factor which they found in milk. In searching for this factor they made a still further discovery for on fractioning the milk they soon learned that the unknown factor was distributed in two different parts of the milk, namely in the butter fat and in the protein free and fat-free whey. The absence of either milk fraction was sufficient to prevent growth. The 1911 publication merely described these results without attempting to explain the nature of the growth producing factors but the vitamine hypothesis of Funk naturally suggested to these authors that their two unknown factors might be similar in nature to his beri-beri curative factor and their announcement may be justly considered a point of junction of nutrition theories with the vitamine hypothesis.

The peculiarity of butter fat as a growth stimulus had been considered from another angle by a German worker, Stepp. In 1909 this student of nutrition had tried to estimate the importance of various types of fats in the same way that was later done with proteins, to determine whether, like proteins, the quality of the fats varied in nutritive efficiency. His experiments were also conducted with white rats and the main outlines of his methods and observations were as follows: Rats fed on a bread and milk diet grew normally. If now the bread and milk mixture was extracted with alcohol-ether the residue was found to be inadequate for growth or maintenance. Stepp assumed that this failure could naturally be ascribed to the removal of the fat by the alcohol-ether mixture. To determine the efficiency of different kinds of fats he then proceeded to substitute in combination with the alcohol-ether extracted diet amounts of purified fats corresponding to what was removed by the alcohol-ether. The results were totally unexpected for none of the purified fats substituted were adequate to secure growth! When, however, he evaporated off his alcohol- ether from the extract of the bread and milk and returned that residue to the diet, growth was resumed as before. The conclusion was obvious, viz., that alcohol-ether takes out of a mixture of bread and milk some factor that is necessary to growth and that factor is not fat but something removed by the extraction with the fat. These results led Stepp to suspect the existence of an unidentified factor but he was unable to identify it as a lipoid. He makes the following statement which is now significant: "It is not impossible that the unknown substance indispensable to life goes into solution in the fats and that the latter thereby become what may be termed carriers for these substances." These studies were published between the years 1909 and 1912 and were therefore concurrent with those of Funk and Osborne and Mendel.

But there was still another set of studies that led up to this vitamine work. In 1907 E. V. McCollum began the study of nutrition problems at the Wisconsin Experiment Station. At the time he was especially interested in two papers that had been published just previous to his entrance into the problem. One of these papers by Henriques and Hansen told how the authors had attempted to nourish animals whose growth was already complete on a mixture consisting of purified gliadin (the principal protein from the quantity viewpoint in wheat), carbohydrates, fats, and mineral salts. In spite of the fact that the nitrogen of this mixture was sufficient to supply the body needs, as proved by analysis of the excreta, the animals steadily declined in weight from the time they were confined to this diet. The authors had assumed that the gliadin was deficient in a substance necessary to growth (lysine) but since their studies were begun only after the animals had reached maximum growth they expected that the growth factor would not be necessary. Why had their animals declined in weight?

The second paper that interested McCollum was by Wilcock and Hopkins. These authors carried out experiments similar to those of the paper just cited but using corn protein (zein) in place of gliadin. This protein had already been shown to be deficient in a chemical constituent known as tryptophan. Animals fed on the zein mixture died in a few days but the inexplicable thing was that when the missing tryptophan was added to the diet the animals lived a little longer but finally declined and died. Why?

McCollum wished to answer this "Why?" These experimenters had complied with every known law of nutrition and yet their mixtures failed to nourish the animals. What was lacking? Earlier work at the Station by Professor Babcock suggested an interesting line of attack and in collaboration with Professors Hart and Humphries, McCollum began a series of studies that have become classic contributions to the vitamine hypothesis and brought this worker into the field as one of the most important contributors to the subject. His initial experiments may be briefly summarized as follows: Young heifer calves weighing 350 pounds at the start and as nearly alike in size and vigor as could be obtained were selected as experimental animals. These were divided into groups and fed with rations so made up as to be alike in so far as chemical analysis could determine, but differing in that the sources of the ration were divided between three plants. One group was supplied with a ration obtained entirely from the wheat plant. A second group derived their ration solely from the corn plant. A third from the oat plant and a fourth or control group from a mixture of oat, wheat and corn. By chemical analysis each group received enough of its particular plant to produce exactly the same amount of protein, fat and carbohydrate and all were allowed to eat freely of salt. All groups ate practically the same amount of feed, and digestion tests showed that there was no difference in the digestibility of the different rations. Exercise was provided by allowing them the run of a yard free of all vegetation. It was a year or more before any distinct change appeared in the different groups. At that time the cornfed animals were in fine condition. On the contrary, the wheat-fed group were rough coated, gaunt in appearance and small of girth. The oat-fed group were better off than the wheat-fed but not in so good shape as the corn-fed. In reproduction the corn-fed animals carried their young well. They were carried for the full term and the young after birth were well formed and vigorous. The wheat-fed mothers gave birth to young from three to five weeks before the end of the normal term. The young were either born dead or died within a few hours after birth. All were much under weight. The oat-fed mothers produced their young about two weeks before the normal period. Of four young, so born, one was born dead, two so weak that they died within a day or two and the fourth was only saved by special measures. The young of the oat-fed mothers were of nearly the same size, however, as those of the corn-fed mothers. After the first reproduction period, the mothers were kept on this diet another year and the following year repeated the same process with identical results. During the first milk-producing period the average production per day was 24.03 pounds per day for the corn-fed, 19.38 pounds for the oat-fed, and 8.04 pounds for the wheat-fed. During the second period it was 28.0, 30.1, and 16.1 pounds per day respectively during the first thirty days.

Every chemical means was now employed to determine the causes of these differences and without success. McCollum then decided to attempt to solve the problem by selecting small animals (the rat was used) and experiment with mixtures consisting of purified proteins from different sources, combined with fats, carbohydrates and mineral salts until a clue was obtained to the nature of the deficiencies. His early results in this direction confirmed the results of other investigators, animals lived no longer on these diets than when allowed to fast. What was missing? Up to 1911 the main result of these experiments had been to call attention to the peculiar deficiencies of cereals and especially in mineral salts, but without unlocking the mystery.

These collateral investigations show how in all parts of this country and on the other side of the ocean events were marching toward the same goal. The year 1911 then is a significant epoch, for from this time the various independent efforts began to link up and the next few years carried us far toward the goal.

In 1912 McCollum was working with a mixture consisting of 18 per cent. purified protein in the form of milk curd or casein, 20 per cent. lactose or milk sugar, 5 per cent. of a fat and a salt mixture made up to imitate the salt content of milk. The remainder of that mixture was starch. With this mixture McCollum found that growth could be produced if the fat were butter fat but not if it were olive oil, lard, or vegetable oils of various sorts. Carrying out the lead here suggested he tried egg yolk fats. They proved as effective as butter fat.

I (from _Journ. Biol. Chem._, 1913, xv, 167). This chart shows the effect in period III of the addition of an ether extract of egg, 1 gram being given every other day. The diets for periods I-IV were as follows:

Periods . . . . I II III IV Salt mixture . . . . 6 6 6 6 Casein . . . .
18 18 18 18 Lactose . . . . 20 0 0 0 Dextrin 0 59
74 74 Starch . . . . 31 0 0 0 Agar-agar . . . . 5 2 2 2 Egg
(see above) . . . . 0 0 * 0 *1 gram extract every other day

II and III (from _Journ. Biol. Chem._, 1915, xxiii, 231). These charts show the effect (II) of the addition of as little as 2 per cent wheat embryo as sufficient to secure normal growth when it serves as a supply of the B vitamine. Chart III shows that even when the wheat embryo is increased to 30 per cent it is inadequate for growth unless the A is also present. The diets were as follows:

Dextrin . . . . 69.3 52.8 Salt mixture . . . . . . 3.7 2.6 Butter fat 5.0
0.0 Agar-agar . . . . 2.0 2.0 Casein . . . . 18.0 12.6 Wheat embryo . . . . . .
2.0 30.0]

These results linked up with those of Stepp and Mendel and showed that butter fat and egg yolk fat contained a growth factor which was missing in other fats. McCollum named this the "unidentified dietary factor fat- soluble

A."

In the same year F. G. Hopkins in England announced that the addition of 4 per cent of milk to diets consisting of purified nutrients would convert them into growth producers. This was too small an amount to admit of attributing the cause to milk proteins, fats, carbohydrates, or salts. Hopkins therefore suggested the existence of unknown factors in milk of the type to which he had earlier given the name "accessory factors." This work has recently been repeated by Osborne and Mendel who fail to find the high potency in milk ascribed to it by Hopkins but the latter's work, at that time, was accepted without question and became the impetus to important discoveries.

Mendel and Osborne had meanwhile investigated more in detail their milk fractions. They obtained results that confirmed McCollum's findings for butter fat but in addition they showed that by removing all the fat and protein from milk they obtained a residue which played an important part in growth stimulation and that this factor was different from the salts present in the mixture. This specially prepared milk residue they called protein-free milk.

The next few years are a melting pot of investigations. They included some sharp controversies over nomenclature and many apparently contradictory conclusions based on what we now know to be insufficient data. The principal outcome was the identification of the yeast and rice polishing substance with the factor carried by protein-free milk. On the basis of these results Funk put forward the idea that McCollum's butter-fat and egg-yolk factor was merely vitamine which clung to the fats as an adulterant. It was soon shown, however, that butter fat could be obtained that was absolutely free of nitrogen and still be stimulatory to growth. It was therefore clear that whatever the factor present it could not be the Funk vitamine. From out of the smoke of this controversy came an ultimate explanation that was very simple. There were two factors instead of one. McCollum did not discover the presence of the Funk vitamine in his mixtures at first because it was carried by the lactose and he did not know it. Finally, to cut a long story very short, these two factors or vitamines were both found to be essential to growth and in the feeding mixtures that had been used were distributed as follows

Vitamine A Fat-soluble Non-antineuritic Present in butter fat and egg-yolk fat

Vitamine B (_Funk's vitamine_) Water-soluble Antineuritic Present in protein-free milk, ordinary lactose, yeast and rice polishings

These four charts all show the power of sources of the A vitamine to bring about recovery after failure on diets lacking that vitamine.

I (from _Journ. Biol. Chem._, 1913-14, xvi, 423). In this group the diet consisted of the following percents: Protein, 18; starch, 26; protein free milk, 28; lard, 28. In the part of the periods marked butter, 18 per cent of butter was substituted for an equal amount of lard.

II (from _Jour. Biol. Chem._, 1913, xv, 311). Shows recovery on addition of butter fat to a diet containing all the nutrients and artificial protein free milk. These diets contained the following percents: Protein, 18; lactose, 23.8; starch, 26; milk salts, 4.2; total fats, 28.

III (from _Journ. Biol. Chem._, 1915, xx, 379). These show the effect of various sources of vitamine A such as egg fat, butter fat and oleomargarine. The broken line parts show the failure of laboratory prepared lard to better the commercial lard of the basal diet and the crossed lines the immediate effect when a true source of vitamine A was added. Basal diet: Protein, 18, protein free milk, 28; starch, 24-29; lard, 7-28; other fats, 0-18.

IV (from _Journ. Biol. Chem._, 1913-14, xvii, 401). This chart shows the failure of almond oil as a source of vitamine A and the prompt recovery when butter fat or cod-liver oil was used. Basal diet: Edestin, 18; starch, 28; protein free milk, 28; lard, 8; almond oil or butter fat or cod-liver oil, 18.]

With these points cleared up each nutrition investigator returned to an analysis of his foodimixtures and proceeded to the location in sources of the various factors. The years 1912-1918 are mainly contributory to further knowledge of the properties of these two vitamines, their reactions, source, behavior, etc. In 1912, however, Holst and Frilich began a study of scurvy that was to culminate later by adding to the list a new member of the family, viz., vitamine "C."

The disease of scurvy and its prevention by use of orange juice potatoes, etc., was a well known phenomenon and to the curative powers of lime juice we owe the name "lime-juicers" as a synonym for the British merchant marine.

Following his discovery of vitamine as the preventative substance to beri-beri, Funk had outlined a theory of "avitaminoses" as the responsible cause of several other types of diseases, including scurvy, rickets, pellagra, and beri-beri. In other words, he suggested that the etiology of these diseases would be found to lie in the lack of the vitamine factors. His views at the time were largely hypothetical since the only one of his avitaminose then demonstrated was beri-beri, but the hypothesis attracted attention and developed a new method of study as it had in matters of normal nutrition.

Between 1907 and 1912 Holst and Frilich had made exhaustive studies of the causes of scurvy and had reached the conclusion that its cause was due to the absence of some factor, admittedly unknown, but as strongly indicated as in the case of beri-beri. Holst pointed out that a guinea pig restricted to a diet of oats became affected with scurvy. McCollum as well as others were attracted to this problem and in 1918 McCollum stated that scurvy was not due to a lack of a dietary factor but to the absorption from the intestine of the poisonous products resulting from abnormal decomposition of the food and especially of protein food. He studied the guinea pig on an oat diet and drew the conclusion that while it does induce scurvy this result is not due to the absence of any specific factor in the oat diet. He showed that while the oat kernel contains all the chemical elements and complexes necessary for the growth and health of an animal these elements are not in suitable proportions. It lacks certain mineral salts and its content of the "A." vitamine is too low to permit oats alone to give satisfactory growth results. Furthermore its proteins are not of as good quality as those of milk, eggs, and meat. By merely supplementing the oat diet with better protein, salts, and a growth promoting fat, he reported that a guinea pig could be developed normally without further addition and that therefore it was impossible to show that any unknown factor was responsible for the scurvy symptoms. McCollum also reported that the guinea pig could develop scurvy even when his diet was supplemented with fresh milk and since milk was a complete food it followed that the cause of the disease must be sought outside of dietary factors.

Examination of guinea pigs that died of scurvy showed that the cecum was always full of putrefying feces. This observation suggested that the mechanical difficulty these animals have in removing feces from this part of the digestive tract might have something to do with the disease. McCollum and his workers were confirmed in their views by the excellent results that followed the use of a mineral oil as a laxative. Another piece of evidence they gave for their views was that when animals were fed on oats and milk the onset of the scurvy could be delayed by merely adding the cathartic, phenolphthalein, to the mixture. They met the argument of the curative power of orange juice by preparing an artificial juice of citric acid, inorganic salts and cane sugar and showing that this synthetic mixture which held only known substances was capable of protecting animals from scurvy over a long period of time. Without going further into the evidence presented by these workers McCollum was sufficiently convinced of the correctness of his own views to not only state them in his researches but to set them forth at length for public information in his book entitled The Newer Knowledge of Nutrition. In spite of all this evidence his views failed to convince the holders of the vitamine hypothesis. Harden and Zilva and Chick and Hume in England freely criticised his conclusions because whole milk was used in his experiments and no attention paid to the amounts eaten. It was then well known that if enough whole milk is eaten scurvy will not develop. Cohen and Mendel autopsied normal guinea pigs and found that the cecum was nearly always full of feces. On the other hand in autopsies of many pigs dead from scurvy only one-fourth were found to show the impaction of feces claimed by McCollum as cause of the disease. Milk is constipating to guinea pigs. Large amounts of milk should therefore have increased scurvy if the cause stated by McCollum was the real one. On the contrary large amounts of milk prevented scurvy and small doses permitted it to develop. The use of coarse materials as a preventative of constipation failed to prevent scurvy onset. Hess and Unger found that cod-liver oil and liquid petrolatum prevented constipation but failed to prevent scurvy.

The attack on the McCollum view continued from various quarters. Chick and Hume in England examined his grain and milk fed series and showed that those receiving much milk and little grain recovered while those on the reverse diet died. They held that all guinea pigs with scurvy become constipated regardless of the diet. They gave large quantities of dried vegetables well cooked in water, in order to provide bulk, but this did not prevent scurvy and neither did the use of mineral oil. Hess found that in infants with scurvy there is a history of constipation but that while potatoes which are not laxative cure scurvy, malt soups which are laxative permit its development. He found that scurvy in infants is relieved by amounts of orange juice entirely too small to have a marked laxative action and was unable to secure cures with McCollum's artificial orange juice. The most convincing argument was the discovery that orange juice administered intravenously still exerted a curative action which could not in any way be laid to its effect on constipation.

To these attacks McCollum's co-worker, Pitz, suggested a new hypothesis. It was well known that in rats and man the intestinal flora can be changed from a putrefactive form to a non-putrefactive type by feeding milk sugar or lactose. If this were true, as was admitted by all, and the scurvy due to the absorption of putrefactive products, this absorption might still be the causal factor whether constipation was present or absent. To determine this point he fed his guinea pigs on oatmeal to which he added a carbohydrate diet. When the carbohydrate was lactose he was able to cure and prevent scurvy. This evidence was not considered convincing, however, since in his experiments milk was given freely. Furthermore, Cohen and Mendel demonstrated that in their experiments pure lactose neither prevented nor cured scurvy while Harden and Zilva could find no antiscorbutic value in either cane sugar, fructose, or sirup. These authors believed and stated that Pitz's results were entirely attributable to the free use of raw milk.

As this milk factor came increasingly to the attention in the controversy it was natural that students began to reexamine this product more carefully. The vitamine advocates at first believed that its potency as an antiscorbutic was of course due to the vitamines already found present therein, viz., the "A" or the "B." But there began to be difficulties with this view. Hess found that eggs and cod-liver oil, both rich in "A" were of no value as scurvy cures. These experiments eliminated the "A" as the curative factor. Cohen and Mendel used a mixture of yeast and butter in their experiments without success. These experiments threw doubt on the "B" as a curative factor. Studies in heated milk had also shown that the scurvy curing power was destroyed by such procedures as heating and that pasteurized milk was not as good as raw milk. This heating on the other hand did not destroy the antineuritic power of the milk nor its growth- stimulating properties. The combined result of all these studies was to eliminate both the "A" and the "B" as the vitamines with antiscorbutic power without suggesting a better hypothesis than McCollum's.

Gradually, however, it became evident that while scurvy is not prevented by either of these vitamines Funk's hypothesis and Holst and Frilich's experimental evidence was correct and McCollum's view wrong. The answer lay in the discovery of a third vitamine, water-soluble like "B" but otherwise of entirely different behavior and properties. J. C. Drummond of England finally suggested its inclusion in the family and the name water- soluble "C." As soon as its presence was admitted and its properties roughly determined the way was opened to development of the antiscorbutic vitamine hypothesis and that has now proceeded as rapidly as in the other fields. During the past year many contributions have been made in this field. Sherman, La Mer, and Campbell have recently published results that have taught us much about the measurement of this new member and its manipulation in experimental study of scurvy.

The year 1920, then, has brought us to a recognition of at least three members of the family. Still more recently another deficiency disease has been under investigation and Hess has found in cod-liver oil a remedy for rickets that he cannot believe owes its efficiency to the "A" type. Mellanby of England believes the "A" vitamine is the preventive factor in this disease but Hess's results at least suggest the possibility that the antirachitic vitamine may be separate and distinct from any of those yet named, possibly vitamine "D?" Others are beginning to doubt the identity of the rat growth promoter and the beri-beri curing complexes and feel that the "B" itself may be the name of a group instead of a single entity. All of these features make one feel uncertain to say the least, as to the limits of this vitamine family or of the future possibilities but enough has been given to indicate the historical development to date and we can now turn to more special features of the subject and their bearing on every day affairs.

CHAPTER II

THE ATTEMPTS TO DETERMINE THE CHEMICAL NATURE OF A VITAMINE

The discovery of the existence of an unknown substance is naturally a stimulation to investigation of its nature. In the case of the vitamines we have many researches to this end but extremely meagre results. We are today actually no nearer the goal of identification than we were in 1911 when Funk published his studies on the beri-beri curing type. In brief, we do not know what a vitamine is. Nevertheless, it will be of interest to the student to review the attempts that have been made to isolate these substances for such attempts must furnish the starting point for further studies and their description will help to make clear the nature of the problem involved.

The most extensive investigations have dealt with the first type discovered, namely the vitamine "B" or Funk antineuritic type. In 1911 Cooper and Funk found that the alcoholic extract of rice polishings could be precipitated with phosphotungstic acid and that this procedure permitted them to obtain a fraction that was particularly potent and free from proteins, carbohydrates, and phosphorus. Funk carried this investigation farther and fractioned the phosphotungstic acid precipitate with silver nitrate, following the usual procedure for separating nitrogenous bases. From the silver-nitrate baryta fraction he obtained a crystalline complex melting at 233. to which he gave the formula $C_{17}H_{20}O_{7}N_{2}$. This substance was curative for pigeons and the fractioning process was applied by him to yeast and other foodstuffs with similar results. From these results Funk believed the vitamine to belong to a class of substances known as the pyrimidine bases. Later, when working with Drummond, Funk was forced to admit that his crystalline complex was not the pure substance, as analysis showed that it contained large amounts of nicotinic acid. His product might well be considered as nicotinic acid contaminated with vitamines.

Suzuki, Shimamura and Odake also used the phosphotungstic precipitation method and claimed to have prepared the crystalline antineuritic substance which they called oryzanin in the form of a crystalline picrate. Drummond and Funk repeated this work, but were unable to confirm the Japanese results. A group of British chemists (Edie, Evans, Moore, Simpson and Webster) obtained an active fraction from yeast and succeeded in separating this into a crystalline basic member belonging to the pyrimidine group which they called torulin.

None of these three preparations have stood the test of analysis however and their curative properties seem to lie in their greater or less contamination with the actual substance, whatever it is. Numerous modifications of the fundamental method for extracting the substance have been planned and executed. Funk for example has shown that if the phosphotungstic precipitate is treated with acetone it is possible to separate it into an acetone soluble and an acetone-insoluble fraction and that the curative fraction is in the latter. McCollum has reported that while ether, benzene and acetone cannot be used to extract the B vitamine from its source, benzene, (and to a slight extent acetone) will dissolve the vitamine if it is first deposited from an alcohol extract on dextrin. These observations have not yielded any further clew to the nature of the substance.

Recently Osborne and Wakeman have proposed a modification which yields a concentrate of high potency. Their method is to add fresh yeast to slightly acidified boiling water and continue the boiling for about five minutes. This process coagulates the proteins that are present and permits their removal by filtration. The protein-free filtrate appears to contain all of the vitamine originally present in the yeast but attempts to precipitate the vitamine fractionally from the evaporated filtrate by means of increasing concentration of added alcohol has been only partially successful. The method however yields a concentrated extract, and Harris has made use of this process to prepare tablets for medicinal purposes.

Seidell and Williams some time ago devised a procedure which seemed to give promise of good results. Their discovery was that when a filtrate from autolysed yeast is prepared, rich in the vitamine, and is shaken with a specially activated fuller's earth (the preparation produced by Lloyd and known as Lloyd's reagent has this power) in a proportion of 50 grams to the liter of extract the vitamine is absorbed by the earth and when the latter is filtered off it carries the vitamine with it. In their process they shake the mixture for about one-half hour and then remove the earth by filtration. Analysis of the yeast liquor after the extraction shows it to contain practically the same solids as originally present but to have lost practically all its vitamine. The latter is firmly attached to the earth and repeated washing with water fails to remove any appreciable amount of vitamine from it. Furthermore the vitamine-activated fuller's earth retains its active vitamine properties for at least a period of two years. Large amounts of the vitamine can be accumulated in this way and when fed to animals or infants the vitamine is liberated physiologically and produces the usual effects of a vitamine extract. When this discovery was made the discoverers thought that in the fuller's earth they had a means for arriving at the identification of the substance but attempts to recover the vitamine from the earth developed unexpected difficulties. Acids were found to split it off but they also split off aluminium compounds and left an impure mixture little better than the original extract for study. By using a dilute alkali they were able to obtain the substance without aluminium contaminations and by this method they actually obtained some microscopic fibrous needles which were curative. These needles however on recrystallization resulted in the production of a compound contaminated with adenin or rather in adenin contaminated with the curative substance and on standing for some time the adenin crystals gradually lost their curative power. These results led Williams to suggest an interesting hypothesis. By experiments conducted with the hydroxy-pyridines he believed that he had demonstrated a relation between tautomerism or changed space relations in these sort of substances and curative properties. He states his view as follows:

The vitamines contain one or more groups of atoms constituting nuclei in which the curative properties are resident. In a free state these nuclei possess the vitamine activity but under ordinary conditions are spontaneously transformed into isomers which do not possess an antineuritic power. The complementary substances or substituent groups with which these nuclei are more or less firmly combined in nature exert a stabilizing and perhaps otherwise favorable influence on the curative nucleus, but do not themselves possess the vitamine type of physiological potency. Accordingly it is believed that while partial cleavage of the vitamines may result only in a modification of their physiological properties, by certain means disruption may go so far as to effect a complete separation of nucleus and stabilizer, and if it does so will be followed by a loss of curative power due to isomerism. The basis for the assumption that an isomerization constitutes the final and physiologically most significant step in the inactivation of a vitamine is found in the studies of synthetic antineuritic products. This assumption is supported by evidence ... of the existence of such isomerism in the crystalline antineuritic substances obtainable from brewer's yeast.

According to this view the active adenin obtained was not a contamination but an inactive isomer of the active substance. The hydroxy-betaines which Williams prepared in defense of his theory have been repeatedly tested but have in general failed to confirm his view which stands today as an interesting suggestion but without confirmatory evidence. Other attempts by these authors to fraction their alkaline extract of fuller's earth have been unsuccessful. It is of course well known that alkali acts upon the vitamine destructively. On this account the authors of this method operate as rapidly as possible and restore the alkali extract to a neutral or acid medium quickly. The aqueous extract obtained from the earth in this manner has been shown by Seidell to possess only about one-half of the vitamine originally present in the solid but the vitamine in it is shown to be fairly stable. Seidell has not yet determined how long it remains so. Attempts to recover the vitamine from such aqueous solutions have however totally failed to date. To quote Seidell from a recent publication:

By careful evaporation of the solution the products successively obtained show more or less activity by physiological tests but in no case does the resulting material possess the appearance or character which a pure product would be expected to show. Solvents such as benzene, ethylacetate and chloroform fail to effect a separation of active from inactive material. In all fractioning operations the vitamine tends to distribute itself between the fractious rather than to become concentrated in one or the other.

The difficulties encountered by Seidell in this fractioning study have led him to adopt Walsche's idea that vitamines are of the nature of enzymes and hence present all the difficulties of identification and isolation of those substances.

During 1920 Myers and Voegtlin attacked the problem. They have made a discovery that is useful as a separatory process. This that the "B" vitamine is not only soluble in water, but also olive oil and in oleic acid. By shaking an autolysed yeast extract with those solvents in the proportion of 1 cc. of solvent to which 4 cc. of extract the vitamine passes into the oil. When this activated oil is filtered and taken up with eight to ten volumes of ether it in possible to concentrate the ether extract in vacuo and extract from it with 0.1 per cent. HCl an active fraction. Aside from this observation however nothing further has been reported and the possibility of this method of concentration remains yet to be exploited. They did report other methods of fractioning which yielded crystals but failed to produce a pure active substance. Those results add nothing to what has been previously reported except a new method of fractioning and the elimination of the following substances as contributing nothing to vitamine activity (purines, histidine, proteins and albumoses). The crystals they obtained wore contaminated with histamine.

The World War has prevented full knowledge of the work of the German investigators but nothing has appeared that indicates any progress in this field with the exception of a paper by Aberhalden and Schaumann and some work by Hofmeister. The Aberhalden paper yields no new data of any moment and no active substances in pure condition are reported. The reports from Hofmeister are to the effect that he has isolated a very active solution belonging to the pyrimidine series. It yields a crystalline hydrochloride and double salt with gold chloride and has given it the formula $C_5H_{11}NO_2$.

The author ban recently been able to obtain a concentrate vitamine from an extract of alfalfa or autolysed yeast with the aid of a carbon specially activated by McKee of Columbia University for the adsorption of basic substance. This adsorbent has been found quite as effective as the fuller's earth and it is possible to recover the vitamine from the carbon with treatment by acid. Glacial acetic and heat are especially favorable for this process. The study of this concentrate has not, however, yet reached a stage where it contributes any real data on the subject but merely provides another method for forming concentrates.

If we were to characterize the present status of the search for the "B" type it might be said to have resolved itself into obtaining concentrates of high potency as the first step in the process and this type of investigation is now going on in many laboratories.

If the data is then meagre in the field of the "B" vitamine it is still more limited in the case of the "A" and the "C." One of the earliest difficulties encountered in the study of the "A" vitamine was the failure of fat solvents to extract the material from its richest vegetable sources. If butter or egg yolk is extracted with ether, the fat obtained is rich in the "A" vitamine. If, however, ether-extraction is applied to green leaves or seeds it removes the oils but these oils contain little or no vitamine. Pressing methods also fail to remove the substance from vegetable sources. For example, if we press or extract cotton seed we obtain the oil but the vitamine is retained in the press cake. McCollum suggested the following explanation for this behavior. His idea is that the "A" vitamine while soluble in fat is so bound up in the vegetable source that extraction methods fail to loosen it. When these vegetables are eaten the vitamine is set free in the process of digestion and being fat-soluble passes into solution in the animal fats. Hence, when these fats contain it in solution, they retain it in the process of extraction while, lacking this separatory process, ether fails to loosen it from the vegetable binding. Recently, however, Osborne and Mendel have presented data in regard to this binding and shown that if for ether we substitute an ether-alcohol mixture the removal of the "A" with the fat is fairly complete even from vegetable sources. They advance the idea that preliminary treatment with alcohol is a process which will materially assist in breaking the attachment of the vitamine and render its removal with the fat solvent effective. Butter-fat rich in the "A" vitamine has been conclusively shown to be free of nitrogen and phosphorus and it is generally assumed that the "A" vitamine is a nitrogen-free and phosphorus free compound. Further than that however we know nothing of its nature.

Concerning the "C" we know only that it is like the "B," water-soluble and we know somewhat of its properties, but nothing of its chemical nature.

One of the greatest difficulties still encountered in the study of chemical fractions is the delay in identification of the active portion. For this purpose we must rely on tests that are far from delicate and time-consuming to a degree. As a result the study of only a few fractions must extend over long periods of time with all the cumulation of difficulties in the way of change in material, etc. that this delay implies. An idea of these difficulties can best be obtained by a review of our present methods for vitamine testing and these methods constitute the subject matter of the next chapter.

CHAPTER III

THE METHODS USED IN TESTING FOR VITAMINES

It will be evident that in the absence of exact tests for a substance which is unknown chemically the problem of detecting its presence must be a matter of indirect evidence. When a chemist is presented with a solution and asked to determine the presence or absence of lead in that solution he knows what he is seeking, what its properties are and how to proceed to not only determine its presence but to measure exactly the amount present. No such possibility is present in a test for vitamines, but this lack of knowledge as to the vitamine structure has not left us helpless. We do know enough of its action to permit us to detect its presence and the technique that has been developed for this purpose is now well standardized and involves no mysteries beyond the comprehension of the layman. In the present chapter is outlined the development of vitamine testing together with a discussion of some of the deficiencies and the problems for the future that these deficiencies suggest.

When Casimir Funk made his original studies of the chemical fractions of an alcohol extract of rice polishings he utilized a discovery of the Dutch chemist Eijkman. We have already referred to this discovery, viz., that by feeding polished rice to fowls or pigeons they could be made to develop a polyneuritis which is identical in symptoms and in response to the curative action of vitamine, to the beri-beri disease. A normal pigeon can be made to eat enough rice normally to develop the disease in about three weeks. The interval can be somewhat shortened by forced feeding. As soon as the symptoms develop the bird is ready to serve as a test for the presence or absence of the antineuritic vitamine. If at this time we have an unknown substance to test it can be administered by pushing down the throat or mixed with the food or an extract can be made and administered intravenously. If the dose is curative, the bird will show the effect by prompt recovery from all the symptoms of the disease in as short a time as six to eight hours. Such a procedure provides a qualitative test which can be made roughly quantitative by varying the dosage until an amount, just necessary to cure the bird in a given time is found and then expressing the vitamine content of the food in terms of this dosage, in such an experiment the value is obviously based on the curative powers of the vitamine source. Another way of applying the test is to determine just how much of the unknown must be added to a diet of polished rice to prevent the onset of polyneuritic symptoms. Such a determination will give the content in terms of preventive dosage. Both methods have been extensively applied and the following tables compiled from the Report of the British Medical Research Committee illustrate both the method and some of its results:

_Minimum daily ration that must be added to a diet of polished rice to prevent and to cure polyneuritis in a pigeon of 300 to 400 grams in weight.

The weights are given in terms of the natural foodstuff._

AMOUNT NECESSARY FOR PREVENTION	FOODSTUFFS TESTED	AMOUNT NECESSARY FOR DAILY CURE
grams		grams
1.5	Wheat germ (raw)	2.5
2.5	Pressed yeast	3.0-6.0[1]
3.0	Egg yolk	60.0[2]
20.0	Beef muscle	140.0[2]
3.0	Dried lentils	20.0[2]

[Footnote 1: Autolysed.] [Footnote 2: Alcohol extract.]

These values illustrate both the method and its value in comparing sources. Unfortunately experience has shown that polyneuritis is amenable to other curative agents to a greater or less extent and it is difficult to be sure whether the curative or preventive dose represents merely the vitamine content of the unknown or is the sum of all the factors present in the curative or preventive material. In comparing the value of different chemical fractions it probably gives a fair enough basis for evaluating their relative power but it is not entirely satisfactory as a quantitive measure of vitamine content.

In America the comparison of vitamine content has been largely based on feeding experiments with the white rat. No other animal has been so well standardized as this one. Dr. Henry Donaldson of the Wistar Institute of Philadelphia has brought together into a book entitled The Rat the accumulated record of that Institution bearing on this animal. This book provides standards for animal comparisons from every view point; weight relation to age, size and age, weight of organs and age, sex and age and weight, etc. This book together with the experience of many workers as they appear in the literature and especially the observations of Osborne and Mendel have made the rat an extremely reliable animal upon which to base comparative data. The omnivorous appetite of the animal, his ready adjustment to confinement, his relatively short life span, all contribute to his selection for experimental feeding tests. Another important reason for his selection is that being a mammal we may reasonably consider that his reactions to foods will be more typical of the human response than would another type, the bird for example. It is perhaps necessary to sound a warning here, however, and point out the danger of too great faith in this comparability of rat and man or in fact of any animal with man. In the case of the rat he has been found useless for the study of "C" vitamine for the simple reason that rats do not have scurvy. In general however his food responses to the vitamines, at least of the "A" and "B" types, have proved, so far as they have been confirmed by infant feeding, to be reasonably comparable.

Provided with the experimental animal the next step was to devise a basal diet which should be complete for growth in every particular except vitamines. Such basal diets have been a process of development. The requirements for such a diet are the following factors:

1. It must be adequate to supply the necessary calories when eaten in amounts normal to the rat's consumption.

2. It must contain the kinds of nutrients that go to make up an adequate diet and in the percents suitable for this purpose.

3. It must contain proteins whose quality is adequate, for growth, i.e., which contain the kinds and amounts of amino acids known to fulfil this function.

4. It must be digestible and palatable.

5. It must be capable of being supplemented by either or both vitamines in response to the particular test it is devised to meet and when both are present in proper amounts it must produce normal growth and serve as a control.

The cages being bottomless are readily cleaned. They are set on circles of wire mesh over galvanized iron funnels permitting urine and feces to pass through. A second screen over the collecting cup and of fine mesh separates the feces from urine and also collects scattered food.]

In building up such a diet many experiments have been combined and thanks largely to the efforts of Osborne and Mendel and McCollum in this country, we have a thoroughly standardized procedure even extending to types of cages and care best suited to normal growth and development. For clearer appreciation of the nature of these diets and their preparation we have summarized in the following pages the combinations used by the principal contributors to the subject in this country.

The dial is so made that it can be set to counterbalance the weight of the cage and the weights read directly. This is also used for weighing food.]

It is at once obvious from the table that the testing value of these basal diets demands the absence of the two vitamines in the protein, carbohydrates and fat fractions. To make sure of this absence various methods have be devised to attain the maximum purity. The authors recommend the following procedure:

a. To purify the casein or other protein used. Boil the protein three successive times (it is assumed that the original is already as pure as it is possible to obtain it by the usual methods of preparation) for an hour each time, with absolute alcohol, using a reflux condenser to prevent loss of alcohol. Filter off the alcohol each time by suction. This process will take off all the adherent fat and hence all the "A" vitamine that might be present. The casein is then dried and ready for use. In certain experiments the authors use meat residues instead of a single protein. This they prepare as follows: Fresh lean round of beef is run through a meat chopper and then ground to a paste in a Nixtamal mill, stirred into twice its weight of water and boiled a few minutes. The solid residue is then strained, using cheese cloth, pressed in the hydraulic press and the cake stirred into a large quantity of boiling water. After repeating this process of washing with hot water the extracted residue is rapidly dried in a current of air at about 60. This dried residue may then be further purified with the absolute alcohol treatment as described for casein.

b. To purify the carbohydrate they treat starch in exactly the same way as the casein.

c. To purify the lard. This is melted and poured into absolute alcohol previously heated to 60., cooled over night and filtered by suction. This process is repeated three times and the resulting solids dried in a casserole over a steam bath.

d. When butter fat is used to provide a source of "A" vitamine it is prepared as follows: Butter is melted in a flask on a water bath at 45. and then centrifugated for an hour at high speed. This results in a separation of the mixture into three layers: (a) Clear fat, containing the "A" vitamine and consisting of 82 to 83 per cent glycerides. This is siphoned off and provides the butter fat named in the diets, (b) An aqueous opalescent layer consisting of water and some of the water-soluble constituents of the milk. This is rejected. (c) A white solid mass consisting of cells, bacteria, calcium phosphate and casein particles. This is also rejected.

Osborne and Mendel's diet

(Figures give the per cent of each ingredient in the diet)

INGREDIENTS	VITAMINE FREE			CONTAINING A ONLY			
	I	II	III	IV	V	VI	VII
Purified protein as casein, lactalbumin, edestin, egg albumin, etc.	18.0	18.0		18.0	18.0	18.0	
or Meat residue				19.6			19.6
Carbohydrates in the form of: Starch	29.5	54.0	52.4	29.5	54.0	54.0	52.4
Sucrose				15.0			15.0
Fat in the form of: Lard	30.0	24.0	24.0	15.0	15.0	15.0	15.0
Butter fat							15.0
Egg yolk fat	9.0		9.0				9.0
Cod liver oil							
Salts in the form of: Salt mixture I	2.5		2.5				
or Artificial protein-free milk (Mixt. IV)		4.0	4.0		4.0	4.0	4.0
or Protein-free milk							
Roughage in the form of: Agar-agar				5.0			5.0
Total	100.0	100.0	100.0	100.0	100.0	100.0	100.0

INGREDIENTS	A ONLY	CONTAINING B ONLY

```
                                    |            |
_____|_____|_____
_____ | | | | | | | | VIII| IX | X | XI | XII | XIII| XIV Purified protein as
casein, | | | | | | | lactalbumin, edestin, egg | | | | | | | albumin, etc. . . . . . . .
| 18.0|18.0 | 18.0| 18.0| | 18.0| 18.0 or Meat residue . . . . . | | | | | 19.6| |
| | | | | | | Carbohydrates in the form of: | | | | | | | Starch . . . . . . . . . . . |
45.0| 45.0| 29.5| 54.0| 52.4| 26.0| 29.0 Sucrose . . . . . . . . . . . | | | 15.0| | |
| | | | | | | | Fat in the form of: | | | | | | | | Lard . . . . . . . . . . . | 15.0| 27.0|
30.0| 24.0| 24.0| 28.0| 25.0 Butter fat . . . . . . . . . | | | | | | | Egg yolk fat . . . . . . . .
| | | | | | | Cod liver oil . . . . . . . . | 18.0| 6.0| | | | | | | | | | | Salts in the
form of: | | | | | | | Salt mixture I . . . . . . . | | | 2.5| | | | or Artificial protein-
free | | | | | | | milk (Mixt. IV) . . . . . . | 4.0| 4.0| | 4.0| 4.0| | or Protein-free
milk . . . | | | | | | 28.0| 28.0 | | | | | | | Roughage in the form of: | | | | | |
|   Agar-agar   .  .   .    .    .    .   .   .    .   .  |  |   |   5.0|   |   |   |
_____|____|____|____|____|____|____|__
___|_____ | | | | | | Fed Daily | | |_____"B"
vitamine in the form of: | | | | | | | | | | | 0.2 | 0.4 | 0.2 | 0.04| | | | to |
gram| to | gram| Dried brewers' yeast | | | 0.6 | | 0.6 | | | | | gram| |
gram|                                                                      |
_____|____|____|____|____|____|____|__
___|_____   |  |  |  |  |  |  |   Total   .   .    .    .    .    .    .    .
|100.0|100.0|100.0|100.0|100.0|100.0|100.0
_____|____|____|____|____|____|____|__
___|_____
```

[Note. Diets I, III and X have been practically discontinued at the present time. Diets II, V and XI are standard. For data on salt mixtures see Osborne, T. B. and Mendel, J. B. The inorganic elements in nutrition, Jour. Biol. Chem. 1918, xxxiv, 131.]

Salt mixture I (after Rohman)

grams Ca_3(PO_4)_2 . . . . . 10.00 K_2HPO_4 . . . . 37.00 NaCl . . . .
20.00 Na citrate . . . . . . 15.00 Mg citrate . . . . . . 8.00 Ca lactate . . . . . . 8.00 Fe
citrate . . . . . . 3.00 _____

Total 100.00

Artificial protein-free milk

grams CaCO_3 . . . . 134.8 MgCO_3 . . . . 24.2 Na_2CO_3 . . . .
34.2 K_2CO_3 . . . . 141.3 H_3PO_4 . . . . 103.2 HCl 53.4
H_2SO_4 . . . . 9.2 Citric acid: H_2O . . . 111.1 Fe citrate: 1.5H_2O . . 6.34
KI . . . . 0.020 MnSO_4 . . . . 0.079 NaF 0.248
K_2Al_2(SO_4)_2 . . . . 0.0245

[N.B.--The ingredients of the artificial protein-free milk are mixed as follows: Making proper allowance for the water in the chemicals the acids are first mixed and the carbonates and citrates added. The traces of KI, MnSO_4, NaF, and K_2Al_2(SO_4)_4 are then added as solutions of known concentration. The mixture is then evaporated to dryness in a current of air at 90 to 100?Centigrade and the residue ground to a fine powder.]

e. When brewers' yeast is used as a source of the "B" vitamine it is first dried over night in an oven at 110 癈. and then subjected to the same purification process as the casein and the starch to remove all trace of the "A."

The reasons for the special precautions just described have arisen from some recent work of Daniels and Loughlin who claim that commercial lard contains enough "A" vitamine to permit rats to grow, reproduce and rear young. The British authorities explain their results as not due to the presence of the "A" vitamine in the lard but to a reserve store in the bodies of the animals. They hold that animals may thus store the "A" vitamine but that apparently they have no storage powers for the "B" that are comparable to it. Osborne and Mendel repeated the experiments described by Daniels and Loughlin, using the purification methods just described, but failed to obtain similar results with either commercial lard or with the purified fraction. They question the validity of the British explanation but at the same time reiterate their belief that even commercial lard contains no "A" vitamine. Whatever the explanation of this particular phenomenon it is important that the basal diet be of purified materials and the methods just described supply the procedure necessary to attain that end.

Before discussing the application of these diets to vitamine testing, attention is called to other basal diets developed by McCollum. This worker has paid especial attention to the deficiencies of the cereal grains and in particular to their salt deficiencies. In his basal diets, we find, as would be expected, special combinations particularly suited to the detection of vitamines in such cereals. McCollum has also devised a method of extracting substances to obtain their "B" vitamine and of depositing it on dextrin. For that reason he uses dextrin instead of starch for his carbohydrate and when he wishes to introduce the "B" vitamine it can be done by his method without having to recalculate the carbohydrate component. His method consists of first extracting the source with ether and discarding this extract. Pure ether will not remove the "B" vitamine. The residue is then reextracted several times with alcohol and the alcohol extracts combined. If now these alcohol extracts are evaporated down on a weighed quantity of dextrin the activated dextrin can be used not only to supply the carbohydrate of the ration but also to carry the "B" vitamine of a given source that is under investigation. McCollum's basal diets and salt mixtures are tabulated in the following chart:

McCollum's basal diets and salt mixtures

| | | | INGREDIENTS | VITAMINE FREE |"A" ONLY | "B" ONLY
_____|_____|_____|_____
_____ | | | | | | Casein . . . . . . |18.0|18.0|18.0|18.0| 18.0 | Same as the vitamine Dextrin . . . . . |57.3|56.3|76.3|78.3| 71.3 | free diet Lactose . . . . . |20.6|20.0| | | | with "B" added Agar . . . . | 2.0| 2.0| 2.0| | 2.0 | as yeasts as Salt mixture 185 . | 2.7| 3.7| 3.7| 3.7| 3.7 | in the Mendel Butter fat . . . . | | | | | | 5.0 | diets or as _____|____|____|____|____|____|_____| extracts carried | on the dextrin. | In the latter | case a given | amount of dextrin Lactose was later discarded when it was shown | carries the to be usually contaminated with the "B" vitamine.| extract of a | known weight | of the source of | the "B"

_____|_____

_____

Cereal   testing   combinations

_____ | | | | | | Wheat . . . . . . |56.6| | | | 70.0 | Wheat embryo . . . | |13.3| | | | Corn . . . . | | |71.3| | | Oats . . . . | | | |60.0| | Skim milk powder . | | | | | | 6.0 Dextrin . . . . . |31.5|76.4|18.0|30.3| 20.0 | 81.0 Salt mixture 185 . | | | 3.7| | | Salt mixture 314 . | | 5.3| | | | Salt mixture 318 . | 6.9| | | | 5.0 | Salt mixture 500 . | | | | 4.7| | Salt mixture ? . . | | | | | | 6.0 Butter fat . . . . | 5.0| 5.0| 5.0| 5.0| 5.0 | 5.0 Agar . . . . | | | 2.0| | | 2.0

_____|____|____|____|____|_____|_____

_____

Salt   mixtures

_____ | | NUMBER   OF   MIXTURES
|_____ | | | | | |

INGREDIENTS	185	314	318	500	211	?
	grams	grams	grams	grams	grams	grams
NaCl	0.173	1.067	1.400	0.5148	0.520	15.00
$MgSO_4$ anhydrous	0.266					1.90
$Na_2HPO_4:H_2O$						
K_2HPO_4	0.954	3.016	2.531	0.3113		34.22
$CaH_4(PO_4)_2:H2O$	0.540			0.276		0.89
Ca lactate	1.300	5.553	7.058	2.8780	1.971	57.02
Ferrous lactate					0.118	
K citrate:H_2O		0.203	0.710	0.5562	0.799	
Na citrate anhydrous						3.70
Ferric citrate			0.100			2.00
Mg citrate						7.00
$CaCl_2$			0.386		0.2569	
$CaSO_4:2H_2O$	0.381	0.578				
Fe acetate						0.100

_____|_____|_____|_____|_____|_____|_____

____|_____

These diets fall as shown, into two classes. The first group correspond to those of Osborne and Mendel and are available for general testing of any unknown. The cereal combinations are so constituted that all deficiencies of salts are covered and the proportions of the cereal are so selected as to provide the right proportions of protein, fat and carbohydrate. By adding enough butter fat to supply the "A" the deficiency in the "B" can be tested and by adjusting the amounts of "B" on the dextrin the cereal deficiency in this vitamine can be obtained. It is obvious that by substituting lard for the butter fat one could use the same mixture properly supplemented with the "B" to determine the "A" deficiencies of the wheat.

The most prominent worker in the field of the "A" vitamine measurement in

America is Steenbock. His basal diets are a combination of those already described.

Steenbock's basal diets per cent Casein (washed with water containing acetic acid) . . . . . 18.0 Dextrin . . . . 73.3 Ether extracted wheat embryo as source of vitamine "B" . . . 3.0 Salt mixture (McCollum, no. 185) . . . . 3.7 Agar 2.0

This was his original basal diet but later he modified it by adopting the McCollum method of carrying his "B" vitamine on the dextrin. This was usually the alcohol extract of 20 grams of wheat embryo. In the following diets the presence of this extract is indicated by the letter (x) following the dextrin.

							INGREDIENTS						
						Casein	18.0	18.0	16.0	18.0	16.0	12.0 Salt 185.	4.0	4.0				Salt 32			4.0	4.0	2.0	2.0 Salt 35					2.5	2.5 Dextrin (x)	76.0	71.0	78.0	57.0		Butter fat		5.0		5.0		Beets				15.0		Potatoes					79.5	Dasheens						83.5 Agar	2.0	2.0	2.0	1.0		

Steenbock's salt mixtures

McCollum's no. 185; see page 44. No. 32 consisted of: grams NaCl . . . . 0.202 Anhydrous $MgSO_4$ . . . . 0.311 K_2HPO_4 . . . . 1.115 Ca lactate . . . . 0.289 $Na_2HPO_4:12H_2O$ . . . . 0.526 $Ca_2H_2(PO_4)_2:H_2O$ . . . . 1.116 Fe citrate . . . . 0.138 No. 35 consisted of: NaCl . . . . 1.00 $CaCO_3$ 1.5

The very nature of these basal diets suggests their use. In general however their utilization for testing purposes is based on the following principles: Since the basal diet supplies all the requirements of a food except the vitamine for which one is testing, it is simply necessary to add the unknown substance as a given percent of the diet and observe the results. If the amount added is small it is assumed that its addition will not appreciably effect the optimum concentrations of nutrients, etc., and for such experiments no allowances are made for the constituents in the unknown. For example let us assume that we wish to test the value of a yeast cake as a source of "B" vitamine. We first select a sufficient member of rats of about thirty days age to insure protection from individual variations in the animals. The age given is taken as an age when the rats have been weaned and are capable of development away from the mother and as furnishing the period of most active growth. These rats are now placed on one of the basal diets which in this case supplies all the requirements except the "B" vitamine. In this experiment any of the diets of Osborne and Mendel or of McCollum will do that have been labelled "A" only. After a week or so on this diet they will have cleared the system of the influence of previous diets and their weight curves will be either horizontal or declining. If now we make the diet consist of this basal diet plus say 5 per cent of yeast cake, the weight curve for the next few weeks will show whether that amount supplies enough for normal growth, comparison being made with the normal weight curve for a rat of that age.

In this method it is assumed that the amount of yeast cake added will not derange the proportions of protein fat, etc., in the basal diet enough to affect optimum conditions in these respects. This is a curative type of experiment. If we wish to develop a preventive experiment the yeast cake may be incorporated in the diet from the first and the amount necessary to prevent deviation from the normal curve determined. Both methods are utilized, the one checking the other. If however the amount of the substance necessary to supply the vitamine required for normal development is large such addition would of course disturb the proportions of nutrients in the normal diet and in that case analysis must be made of the substance tested to determine its protein, fat, carbohydrate and salt content and the basal diet corrected from this viewpoint so as to retain the optimum proportions of these factors. McCollum's cereal testing combinations are illustrative of such methods applied to cereals. Still another method is to add a small per cent. of the unknown and then add just enough of the vitamine tested to make sure that normal growth results. Such a method gives the results in terms of a known vitamine carrier. For example, if we add to a basal diet, sufficient in all but the "A" vitamine (Steenbock's mixture for example), a small per cent of a substance whose content in "A" is unknown and note that growth fails to result we can then add butter fat until the amount just produces normal growth. If now we know just what amount of butter fat suffices for this purpose when used alone we can calculate the part of the butter which is replaced by the per cent of unknown used. To put this in terms of figures will perhaps make the idea clearer. Let us assume that 5 per cent of butter fat in a given diet is sufficient to supply the "A" necessary for normal growth. Assume that the addition of 5 grams of the unknown in 100 grams of the butter-free diet fails to produce normal growth but that by adding 2 per cent of butter fat normal growth is reached. It is obvious under these conditions that 5 grams of the unknown is equivalent in "A" vitamine content to 5 minus 2 grams of butter fat, i.e., is equivalent to 3 grams of butter fat or expressed in per cents the substance contains 0.6 or 60 per cent of the "A" found in pure butter fat.

Experience has shown that it is dangerous to draw conclusions from experiments of too short duration or to base them on too few animals. For complete data the experiments should be carried through the complete life cycle of the rat, including the reproductive period. Otherwise it may turn out that the amount in the unknown while apparently sufficient for normal growths is incapable of sustaining the drain made in reproduction. It is this consideration that makes the accumulation of authoritative data on vitamine contents of foodstuffs so slow and tedious and one of the reasons why we lack satisfactory tables in this particular at present. Osborne and Mendel raise another point of methodology and believe that more accurate results will be obtained if the source of the vitamine is fed separately than if mixed with the basal diet. It is easily possible that since one of the effects of lack of vitamine, especially of the "B" type, is poor appetite, the amount necessary to produce normal growth may be smaller than would appear from results obtained by mixing it in the basal diet. When so mixed the animals do not get enough to maintain appetite and really decline because they do not eat enough rather than because the amount of vitamine given is inadequate to growth. Details of this kind are matters however that particularly concern the experimentalist and as our purpose here is to merely describe the methodology we may perhaps turn now to other types of testing. Before doing so it is perhaps unnecessary to suggest that in all experiments it is important that the food intake consumed be measured. Also that in all such experimentation it is necessary to run controls on a complete diet rather than to rely too much on standard figures. For this latter purpose it is merely necessary to add to the basal diets the "A" as butter fat and the "B" as dried yeast or otherwise to make them complete. Various special mixtures have been tested out for this purpose and the data already presented supplies the information necessary to construct such control diets. Professor Sherman has given me the following as a control diet on which he has raised rats at normal growth rate to the fifth generation:

One-third by weight of whole milk powder. Two-thirds by weight of ground whole wheat. Add to the mixture an amount of NaCl equal to 2 per cent of the weight of the wheat.

A control mixture based on Osborne and Mendel's data would have the following components:

Meat residue 19.6 per cent or casein 18 per cent. Starch 52.4 per cent or 49 per cent. Lard 15 per cent or 20 per cent. Artificial protein-free milk 4 per cent. Butter fat 9 per cent. Dried yeast 0.2 to 0.6 gram, daily.

The preceding description has applied especially to testing for the presence of the "A" or the "B" vitamine. When we come to the methods of testing for the "C" type it is necessary to change our animal. Rats do not have scurvy but guinea pigs do. The philosophy of the tests for the antiscorbutic vitamines then will be identical with that of the polyneuritic methods with pigeons, viz., preventive and curative tests with guinea pigs. The "C" vitamine is especially sensitive to heat and this fact enables us to secure a "C" vitamine-free diet. La Mer, Campbell and Sherman describe their methods as follows:

First select guinea pigs of about 300 to 350 grams weight. Test these with the basal diet until you secure pigs that will eat the diet. Those that will not eat it at first are of no use for testing purposes, for a guinea pig will starve to death rather than eat food he doesn't like. Having secured pigs that will eat they should on a suitable basal diet die of acute scurvy in about twenty-eight days. Their basal diet is as follows:

per cent Skim milk powder heated for two hours at 110. in an air bath to

destroy the "C" vitamine that might be present. . 30 Butter fat . . . .
10 Ground whole oats . . . . 59 NaCl . . . .
1

They claim that when fruit juice addenda are given in minimal protective doses and calculated to unit weight bases, the results are comparable in precision to those of antitoxin experiments.

Old food should be removed every two days and replaced by new, cups being cleaned at the same time. Since this is a scurvy-producing diet its use is obvious. We can let the pig develop scurvy on it and then test the curative powers of the unknown by adding it to the diet or we can add it to the diet from the first and determine the dose necessary to prevent scurvy; or we can determine its effect in terms of a known antiscorbutic such as orange juice by combining it with measured quantities of the orange juice.

There are other diets that have been given for this purpose, e.g., Holst and Frilich induced scurvy by restricting animals to an exclusive diet of cereals (oats or rye or barley or corn). Hess and Unger have used hay, oats and water given ad libitum. All of these and others are subject to criticism on the basis that they are not necessarily adequate in other food factors and may therefore not be fair bases for testing the antiscorbutic powers of the unknown combined with them. Abels has recently shown that scurvy increases susceptibility to infections and believes that the scurvy hemorrhages are brought about by the toxic effects of infection. It is therefore desirable in testing for antiscorbutic power that the basal diet be itself as complete as possible in all factors except the absence of "C."

The study of rickets has already progressed to the stage of calculating rickets-producing diets and the methodology is identical with that for scurvy but this phase of testing still lacks evidence of an antirachitic vitamine and in that uncertainty it is hardly worth while to elaborate these diets here. The British diets are all based on Mellanby's contention that the "A" vitamine is the antirachitic vitamine. This view is not yet accepted by American workers.

In concluding this chapter it is sufficient to state that with our present methodology the accumulation of data for evaluating the vitamine content of various foods is still far from satisfactory and from the chemist's viewpoint the methodology is most unsatisfactory as a means of testing fractional analyses obtained in the search for the nature of the substance, both because of the time consumed in a single test and from the difficulty of using the fractions in feeding experiments when these fractions may themselves be poisonous or otherwise unsuited for mixture in a diet. It is obvious therefore that interest is keen in any possibility of devising a test that will be specific, quick and not require modification of the material tested, because of its unsuitability for feeding. In 1919 Roger J. Williams proposed a method that seemed to offer promise in these respects but which is not yet in the form for quantitative use. It offers promise that entitles it to a special chapter for discussion and the next chapter presents the present status of the so- called yeast test for vitamine "B."

Before turning to this test it is well to call attention here to the importance of the experimental animal. Without the polyneuritic fowls we might never have cured beri-beri, the guinea pig made the solution of the scurvy problem possible and if some way of inducing pellagra in an animal can be devised that scourge may yet be eliminated.

CHAPTER IV

THE YEAST TEST FOR VITAMINE "B"

As far back as the days of Pasteur a controversy arose over the power of yeast cells to grow on a synthetic medium composed solely of known constituents. This controversy hinged on a discussion as to whether these media were efficient unless reinforced with something derived from a living organism. In 1901 Wildier in France published an article in which he showed that extracts of organic matter when added to synthetic media had the power to markedly stimulate the growth of yeast organisms. He did not attempt at the time to identify the nature of this stimulatory substance, but since it was derived from living organisms, he called it "Bios." Soon after the discovery of vitamines the bacteriologists began to discover that they or an analogous factor apparently played a part in the growth of certain strains of bacteria, especially the meningococcus. In 1919 Roger Williams working in Chicago University was struck with the bearing of Wildier's work on the vitamine hypothesis and formed the theory that Wildier's "bios" might be the water-soluble vitamine "B." He proceeded to test out this theory and demonstrated that extracts of substances rich in the "B" vitamine had a marked effect on the stimulation of yeast growth. He developed these experiments and devised a method of comparing the growth of yeast cells when stimulated by such extracts. The results were so striking as to appear to justify his view and he then suggested that his method might be used as a test for the measure of "B" vitamine in a given source. William's method consisted essentially in adding the extract of an unknown substance to hanging drops in which were suspended single yeast cells and observing the rate of growth under the microscope. Soon after, Miss Freda Bachman reinvestigated the problem with various types of yeast and found that practically all types of yeast respond to the stimulation of these "bios" extracts. Her method consisted in the use of fermentation tubes and the stimulatory effect was measured by the amount of CO_2 produced in a given time. By this method she confirmed Williams' view that the "bios" of Wildier was apparently identical with vitamine "B" and that most yeasts require this vitamine for their growth. She also suggested that her method might be made the basis of a test for vitamine content. In 1919 Eddy and Stevenson made extended experiments with these two methods in the attempt to improve the technique and make it serve as a quantitative measure. Their experiments served two purposes, first to bring out certain difficulties in the methods of the two authors from the quantitative viewpoint and the development of a technique to correct these difficulties and secondly to add more data bearing on the specificity of the test. Soon after their publication Funk became interested and coming to the same conclusions as to specificity devised a centrifugating method for measuring the yeast growth. Williams also improved his original method and devised a gravimetric method for the same purpose. From the viewpoint of methodology we now have methods which are suitable as quantitive procedures for determining the effect of extracts of unknown substances on yeast growth and hence if the stimulatory substance is vitamine "B," a means of determining within a space of twenty-four hours the approximate content of stimulatory material in a given source. Since the Funk method is the simplest of these and illustrates the principles involved it will suffice to describe that.

Funk method of yeast test with Eddy and Stevenson modification 1. To a basal diet of 9 cc. of sterile culture medium such as a von Nageli solution [Footnote: von Nageli's solution consists of the following ingredients NH_4NO_3, 1 gram; $Ca_3(PO_4)_2$, 0.005 gram; $MgSO_4$, 0.25 gram dextrose

10.0 grams made up to 100 cc. with distilled water. Other culture media may be used and such combinations will be found in any text on yeasts. They all permit a certain amount of growth but all are apparently stimulated by the addition of vitamine extracts.] in a sterile test tube is added 1 cc. of the sterile, neutral, watery extract of the source of the vitamine. A pure culture of Fleischman's yeast (Funk prefers brewer's yeast) is maintained on an agar slant and twenty-four hours before the test is to be made, a transplant is made to a fresh agar slant. One standardized platinum loopful of the twenty-four hour yeast growth is then used to inoculate the contents of the tube, the tube stoppered with cotton and incubated for from twenty-four to seventy-two hours at a temperature of 31. The seventy-two hour incubation period yields nearly optimum growth for this purpose.

2. At the end of this time the yeasts are killed by plunging the tube in water heated to 80. and maintained at this temperature for fifteen minutes. The contents of the tubes are then poured into a Hopkins centrifuge tube which has a capillary tip graduated in hundredths of a cubic centimeter. After twenty minutes centrifugating at a speed of about 2400 revolutions per minute the yeasts in the solution have all been packed into the tip and the volume can then be read accurately to thousandths of a cubic centimeter (with the aid of a scale and magnifier). With a control tube containing 9 cc. of the sterile media and 1 cc. of distilled water in place of the 1 cc. of extract a comparison can be obtained which is an accurate measure of the stimulatory effect of the extract. If this stimulus is due purely to vitamine it is obvious that this procedure would enable us to compare extracts of known weights of and arrive at comparisons which would be measures of their vitamine content. In other words the procedure is now in a satisfactory form for testing and its value depends merely upon our ability to show that the stimulus given the yeast is due solely to vitamine "B."

The interest of the vitamine student in this test will be easily understood for it is so simple of manipulation and so rapid in producing results that it is the nearest approach to a chemical test of satisfactory nature yet proposed but unfortunately evidence soon began to accumulate to show that the stimulation produced by extracts of various sources is not a matter of pure vitamine. If we plot a curve of stimulation for various dilutions of a given extract we find that the stimulation is not directly proportional to the concentration of vitamine present but is a composite of several factors. The chart derived from experiments by Eddy and Stevenson shows the general nature of this curve. Other experimenters have reached similar results and some have gone so far as to maintain that the stimulation is not due to vitamine "B" at all. It is therefore evident that until this controversy is settled the yeast test cannot be used for the purpose proposed. Our own experiments at present make us still firm in our belief that one of the factors and perhaps the most important factor in the stimulation effect is the vitamine but until we can devise a basal medium that is comparable to that used in rat feeding experiments, i.e., one that contains all the elements for optimum growth of yeasts except vitamine "B" it will be unsafe to draw conclusions from the test as to vitamine content. It may be possible to so treat our extracts as to eliminate from them all other stimuli except the vitamine or to destroy the vitamine in them and thus permit the comparison of an extract with the vitamine destroyed against one in which it is present and thus arrive at the result desired. At any rate all we can say at present is that the yeast test is unreliable as a measure of vitamine content but that if it can be made quantitative its advantages are so great that it is very much worth while to continue work upon it until it is certain that it cannot be made to produce the desired result.

This chart shows the effect of varying concentrations of an alfalfa extract on the growth rate of the yeast cell. The rate of growth was determined after the Funk method by centrifuging the cells after seventy- two hours incubation and measuring the volume in cubic centimeters. The shape of the curve shows that this method will not give comparative results unless the extracts tested are dilute enough for the determinations to fall in the steep part of the curve.]

Another reason for our attention to this test is that if it can be made to show vitamine effect it provides an excellent medium for investigation of vitamine "B" reactions, and a method for studying the effect of the vitamine upon the protoplasm of a single cell.

CHAPTER V

THE SOURCES OF THE VITAMINE

Having now considered the general principles involved in vitamine testing we may justly ask what information they have yielded us in regard to the distribution of the vitamines in nature. If we must include vitamines in our diets it is important to know how to select foods on this basis, hence a classification of them on the ground of vitamine distribution becomes essential. The newness of the subject and the limited tests that have been made as well as the uncertainty residing in the test results make any classifications presented more or less approximations but we present such attempts as have been made, with the understanding that these tabulations are merely guides and not quantitative measurements in the sense that tables giving calorie values of protein, fat and carbohydrate content are. The following table (1) has been freely copied from a report of the British Medical Research Committee to which acknowledgment is hereby given.

TABLE 1

Pages 50 and 61 of the British Medical Research Committee's report

CLASSES OF FOODSTUFFS	VITAMINE "A"	VITAMINE "B"	VITAMINE "C"
Fats and oils:			
Butter	+++	0	
Cream	++	0	
Cod-liver oil	+++	0	
Mutton and beef fat or suet	++		
Lard	0		
Olive oil	0		
Cotton seed oil	0		
Cocoanut oil	0		
Cocoa-butter	0		
Linseed oil	0		
Fish oil, whale oil, herring oil, etc.	++		
Hardened fats (hydrogenated) of animal or vegetable origin	0		
Margarine from animal fat	In proportion to animal fat used		
Margarine from vegetable fat or lard	0		
Nut butters	+		
Meat, fish, etc.:			
Lean meat (beef, mutton, etc.)	+	+	+
Liver	++	++	+
Kidneys	++	+	
Heart	++	+	
Brain	+	+	++
Sweetbreads	+	++	
Fish, white	0	Very slight if any	
Fish fat (salmon, herring, etc.)	++	Very slight if any	
Fish roe	+	++	
Tinned meats	?	Very slight	0
Milk, cheese, etc.:			
Milk, cow's whole raw	++	+	+
Milk, cow's skim	0	+	+
Milk, cow's dried whole	Less than ++	+	Less than +
Milk, cow's boiled whole	?	+	Less than +
Milk, cow's condensed sweetened	+	+	
Cheese, whole milk	+		Less

than | | | + Cheese, skim milk . . . . | 0 | | Eggs, fresh . . . . | ++ | +++ | 0? Eggs, dried . . . . | ++ | +++ | 0? _Cereals, pulses, etc.:_ | | | Wheat, maize, rice (whole germ) | + | + | 0 Wheat, maize, rice germ . . . . | ++ | +++ | 0 Wheat, maize, rice bran . . . . | 0 | ++ | 0 White wheat flour, pure corn | | | flour, polished rice, etc. . | 0 | 0 | 0 Custard powders, egg substi- | | | tutes prepared from cereal | | | products . . . . | 0 | 0 | 0 Linseed, millet . . . . | ++ | ++ | 0 Dried peas, lentils, etc. . . . | | ++ | Pea-flour, kilned . . . . | | 0 | 0 Soy beans, haricot beans . . . | + | ++ | 0 Germinated pulses or cereals . | + | ++ | ++ _Vegetables and fruits:_ | | | Cabbage, fresh, raw . . . . . . | ++ | + | +++ Cabbage, fresh, cooked . . . . | | | + | + Cabbage, dried . . . . . . | + | + |Very slight Cabbage, canned . . . . | | |Very slight Swedes, raw expressed juice . . | | | | +++ Lettuce . . . . | ++ | + | Spinach, dried . . . . | ++ | + | Carrots, fresh, raw . . . . . . | + | + | + Carrots, dried . . . . |Very slight | | Less than | | | + Beetroot, raw, expressed juice | + | + | Potatoes, raw . . . . | | | + Potatoes, cooked . . . . | | | ++ Beans, fresh scarlet runners raw| | | Lemon juice, fresh . . . . . . | | | +++ Lemon juice, preserved . . . . | | | Lime juice, fresh . . . . | | | ++ Lime juice, preserved . . . . . | | |Very slight Orange juice, fresh . . . . . . | | | +++ Raspberries . . . . | | | ++ Apples . . . . | | | + Bananas . . . . | + | + |Very slight Tomatoes, canned . . . . | | | ++ Nuts . . . . | + | ++ | _Miscellaneous:_ | | | Yeast dried . . . . | ? | +++ | Yeast extract and autolysed . . | ? | +++ | 0 Meat extract . . . . | 0 | 0 | 0 Malt extract . . . . | | + in some | | | specimens | Beer . . . . | | 0 | 0 Honey . . . . | | | | | + | _____|_____|_____|_

_____

+++ indicates abundant; ++ relatively large; + present in small amount; 0 absent.

The following table (2) has been compiled from a review of both British and American data and represents a rather more complete classification than the British report. The four plus system has also been used to permit more complete comparisons.

TABLE 2

FOODSTUFF	"A"	"B"	"C"
Meats:			
Beef heart	+	+	?
Brains	++	+++	+?
Codfish	+	+	?
Cod testes	+		
Fish roe	+	++	?
Herring	++	++	?
Horse meat	++	++	
Kidney	++	++	
Lean muscle	0	0	+?
Liver	+	+	+?
Pancreas	0	+++	
Pig heart	+	+	?
Placenta	+		
Thymus (sweetbreads)	0	0	0
Vegetables:			
Beet root	+	+	++
Beet root juice	?	Little	+++
Cabbage, dried	+++	+++	+
Cabbage, fresh	+++	+++	++++
Carrots	+++	+++	++
Cauliflower	++	+++	++
Celery	?	+++	?
Chard	+++	++	?
Dasheens	+	++	?
Lettuce	++	++	++++
Mangels	++	++	?
Onions	?	+++	+++
Parsnips	++	+++	
Peas (fresh)	+	++	+++
Potatoes	0	+++	++
Potatoes (sweet)	+++	++	?
Rutabaga		+++	
Spinach	+++	+++	+++
Cereals:			
Barley	+	+++	?
Bread (white)	+	+?	
Bread (whole meal)	+	+++	?
Maize (yellow)	+	+++	?
Maize (white)	0	+++	?
Oats	+	+++	0
Rice polished	0	0	0
Rice (whole grain)	+	+++	0
Rye	+	+++	0
Corn embryo		+++	
Corn (kaffir)		+++	
Corn (see maize)			
Corn pollen		++	
Malt extract	0	0	0
Wheat bran	0	+	0
Wheat embryo	++	+++	0
Wheat endosperm	0	0	0
Wheat kernel	+	+++	0
Other seeds:			
Beans, kidney		+++	
Beans, navy		+++	0
Beans, soy	+	+++	0
Cotton seed	++	+++	
Flaxseed	++	+++	
Hemp seed	++	+++	
Millet seed	++	+++	
Peanuts	+	++	
Peas (dry)	+?	++	0
Sun flower seeds	+		
Fruits:			
Apples		++	++
Bananas	?	++	++
Grapefruit		+++	+++
Grape juice		+	+
Grapes	0	+	+
Lemons		+++	++++
Limes		++	++
Oranges		+++	++++
Pears		++	++
Raisins		+	+
Tomatoes	++	+++	++++
Oils and fats:			
Almond oil		0	0
Beef fat			

+ | 0 | 0 Butter . . . . | ++++ | 0 | 0 Cocoanut oil . . . . | 0 | 0
| 0 Cod liver oil . . . . | ++++ | 0 | 0 Corn oil . . . . | 0 | 0 | 0
Cotton seed oil . . . . | 0? | 0 | 0 Egg yolk fat . . . . | ++++ | 0 | 0
Fish oils . . . . | ++ | 0 | 0 Lard . . . . | 0 | 0 | 0 Oleo, animal . . . .
| + | 0 | 0 Oleo, vegetable. . . . . | 0 | 0 | 0 Olive oil . . . . | 0 | 0 |
0 Pork fat . . . . | 0? | 0 | Tallow . . . . | 0 | 0 | 0 Vegetable
oils . . . . | 0? | 0 | 0 _Nuts:_ | | | Almonds . . . . | + | +++ |
Brazil nut . . . . | | | +++ | Chestnut . . . . | | | +++ | Cocoanut . . . .
| ++ | +++ | English walnuts . . . . | | +++ | Filbert . . . . | | +++ |
Hickory . . . . | + | + | + Pine . . . . | + | + | + _Dairy
products:_ | | | Butter . . . . | ++++ | 0 | 0 Cheese . . . . |
++ | + | ? Condensed milk . . . . | ++ | + | 0 Cream . . . . | +++
| + | ? Eggs . . . . | ++++ | ++ | 0 Milk powder (skim) . . . . | + |
+++ | +? Milk powder (whole) . . . . . . | +++ | +++ | +? Milk whole . . . .
| +++ | +++ | ++ Whey . . . . | + | +++ | + _Miscellaneous:_ | | |
Alfalfa . . . . | +++ | +++ | ? Blood . . . . | Varies with
source Clover . . . . | +++ | ++++ | ? Honey . . . . | | ++ | 0
Malt extract . . . . | 0 | 0 | 0 Nectar . . . . | 0 | 0 | 0 Timothy . . . .
| ++ | +++ | Yeast, brewers . . . . | 0 | ++++ | 0 Yeast cakes . . . . |
0 | ++ | 0 Yeast extract . . . . | 0 | +++ | 0
_____|_____|_____|__
_____

CHAPTER VI

THE CHEMICAL AND PHYSIOLOGICAL PROPERTIES OF THE VITAMINE

While the chemists have not yet been able to isolate and identify the various vitamines they have succeeded in demonstrating many of the properties of these substances and it is the knowledge of these properties that has enabled us to produce concentrates and conduct tests. Another practical consideration involved in this matter of properties lies in the effect of cooking and commercial methods of food preparation, for not only must we learn where the vitamine resides but how to prevent injury or destruction in our utilization of the source.

The properties of the vitamines may therefore be grouped under two heads: first chemical properties and second physiological properties.

I. CHEMICAL PROPERTIES OF VITAMINE "A"

a. This dietary factor's presence in butter fat and egg yolk fat indicates its solubility in the fat and it would naturally follow that the fat solvents would suffice to remove it with the fats when food sources are treated with such a reagent. Experience has shown however that while ether extraction applied to butter or egg yolk removes the vitamine with the fat this process fails when it is applied to vegetable sources such as cotton seed, corn germ, spinach, lettuce, etc. Neither does the cold or hot press method of oil extraction liberate the vitamine with the oil. Recent experiments by Osborne and Mendel, to which we have previously referred, have shown that preliminary treatment of vegetable sources with alcohol seems to loosen the bond between the source and the vitamine and that when this binding is once loosened subsequent ether extraction will take the vitamine out. That the binding is not difficult to break is shown by the fact that when vegetables are eaten as a source of vitamine the body is able to separate the complex. It is further evident that the body does separate this complex and stores it in animal fat from the experiments with cow feeds and feeding. Milk for example is rich or poor in vitamine according to the supply of the latter in the food given to the cow. The only logical conclusion to be drawn from this observation is that the cow does not synthesize this factor but splits it off from the food source and then, since it is fat soluble, is able to mobilize it in the butter fat of the milk or to a more limited extent in the body fat. This observation as to the dependence of milk content upon food has been confirmed in the case of nursing mothers and suggests the need of especial attention to the diet of the mother during the lactating period.

b. It has been generally assumed that the "A" vitamine is comparatively stable to heat. Sherman, MacLeod and Kramer state that "dry heating at a temperature of 100 癈. with free access of air, only very slowly destroyed fat soluble vitamine." Osborne and Mendel reported that butter fat treated with steam for two hours and a half did not appear to have lost its value as a source of this vitamine. Drummond's earlier work with fish oils and whale oils seemed to confirm this conclusion. Sherman and his co-workers cited above put it this way: "The results thus far obtained emphasize the importance of taking full account of the time as well as the temperature of heating, and of the initial concentration of the vitamine in the food, as well as of the opportunity for previous storage of the vitamine by the test animal." More recent work by Steenbock and his co-workers in America shows that these earlier results are incorrect in the case of butter fat and that twelve hours exposure of butter fat to 100. may, under certain conditions, destroy the efficiency of that substance as a source of the vitamine. Drummond and other English workers have confirmed Steenbock in later experiments. Their work has shown that the presence or absence of oxygen is a factor, which may determine the extent of destruction of the vitamine. Heat alone is of very limited effect but when sources are heated in the presence of oxygen destruction of the A vitamine may be very rapid. Drummond attributes the absence of the A vitamine in lard to the oxidation that takes place in the commercial rendering of this product. We must conclude therefore that while the vitamine may be destroyed by continuous exposure to a temperature of 100 癈. the effect is largely determined by the nature of the process and the way the vitamine is held in the source. Cooking of vegetables therefore will not as a rule result in appreciable destruction of this factor.

c. The process of hydrogenation used in hardening fats appears to completely destroy the vitamine, hence the many lard substitutes now in use must in general be considered "A" vitamine-free regardless of the content of "A" in the fats from which they are derived unless they have been made by blending instead of hydrogenation.

d. Acids and alkalies have apparently little effect on this particular vitamine.

It may be well to state here however that owing to variability in behavior with variation in conditions it is dangerous to draw too general conclusions and until a given source has actually been investigated under specific cooking conditions one should not rely too strongly on analogies based on comparative experiments. This statement applies to all vitamines and presents one of the live subjects of investigation for the cooking schools and the food factories.

e. Little has been learned further about the chemistry of this substance. [Footnote: Since the above was put in type Steenbock has shown that the A vitamine resists saponification and that by saponifying fats which contain the A it may be possible to secure a fraction rich in the vitamine and free of fat.] Butter fat, nitrogen free and phosphorus free is shown to carry the vitamine and it is therefore assumed that the vitamine lacks these elements. It has been claimed that it may be removed from butter fat by prolonged extraction with water but this has not been confirmed by more recent experimenters. Steenbock was the first to call attention to the association of the A vitamine with yellow pigment in plant and animal sources. Butter, egg yolk, carrots, yellow corn contain it while white corn and white roots are less rich in this vitamine. This observation suggested the chemical relation between the vitamine and carotin. It has however been shown by Palmer and others that carotin is not vitamine A. This association of the pigment with the vitamine is therefore apparently a coincidence and this clue has failed as yet to throw light on the chemical nature of vitamine A.

II. THE CHEMICAL PROPERTIES OF VITAMINE "B"

When Funk first studied this substance he conducted all his evaporations in vacuo from fear that higher temperatures would prove destructive. Subsequent investigation however has shown that 100?has very little if any destructive effect if the vitamine is held in acid or neutral solution. Temperatures between 100?and 120?maintained in an autoclave at 15 pounds above normal pressure do tend to slowly destroy the factor. The extent of this destruction also varies with the character of the crude extract. In general, then, there is little fear of injuring this vitamine in ordinary cooking temperatures if the use of alkali is avoided.

The effect of alkali depends upon the temperature to a very marked degree. Osborne has recently reinvestigated this matter and finds that in the presence of a 0.1N solution of alkali at 20 癈. there is very little destruction but that raising the temperature to 90. brings about a marked destruction. Seidell has shown that if the vitamine is absorbed by Lloyd's reagent and this reagent be then extracted with dilute alkali the vitamine passes into the alkaline solution. If the latter is neutralized quickly it is possible to recover most of the vitamine by this method. The effect of alkali becomes of practical importance to the housewife because of certain cooking habits. I refer to the well known practice of adding soda to the water in which vegetables are cooked to soften the vegetable and accelerate the cooking. Daniels and Loughlin in this country investigated this matter and came to the conclusion that this procedure did not produce enough destruction to be dangerous. Later the matter was studied by Chick and Hume in England and these investigators brought out a feature that had perhaps been overlooked in the previous work. Their point was that in ordinary feeding tests the results merely tell whether there is enough vitamine present to produce normal growth. Hence if the substance tested has much vitamine, a large part of it might be destroyed and this fact not appear in the test because enough might still be left to induce normal growth. By reducing the amount tested so that it was just adequate for normal growth and then applying the soda-cooking experimentation they showed that this method of cookery does do serious harm to the vitamine. From the practical point of view it is of course sufficient to show that enough is left after a cooking process to suffice for normal growth when the substance is taken in the portion sizes ordinarily eaten. The effect of alkali deserves more attention on the part of cooks and food preparateurs and we need more data concerning the minimal dose necessary to protect the human animal.

In neutral and acid solution it is perfectly safe to assume little destruction of this vitamin through heat and it is now common practice to boil sources with the extracting reagent and to use the steam bath freely to concentrate and evaporate these extracts. We have recently investigated the effect upon cabbage of cooking in a pressure cooker at eight pounds pressure. The cabbage so cooked, when dried and mixed so as to form 10 per cent of a basal vitamine free diet, yielded all the "B" vitamine necessary to produce normal growth in rats.

The very name of this vitamine indicates its ready solubility in water. It is also soluble in 95 per cent alcohol and either of these extractants may be used to obtain the vitamine. It is not readily soluble in absolute alcohol and 95 per cent is not as good an extractant as water. Substances rich in the vitamine apparently yield the latter more readily if they have first been subjected to autolysis or if the extracting fluid is acidified. Funk was the first to show that yeast produced a greater yield if it was allowed to autolyse before extraction with alcohol. However, Osborne and Wakeman have produced a method of treating fresh yeast by boiling it with slightly acidified water which seem as efficient as autolysis in the yield produced.

The various methods of extraction now in vogue have already been discussed in Chapter II and need not be repeated here. In general it is apparent that to obtain concentrates of high potency it is permissible to employ temperatures of 100. if we will maintain an acid or neutral reaction but that alkali should be avoided wherever possible and when its use is imperative the temperature must be kept below 20 or destruction will result. In applying this rule to cooking operations the results should be determined by direct tests rather than by assumptions based on these generalizations. It should also be noted that the alkalinity of a solution should be determined on the basis of hydrogen ion concentration and not on amount of alkali added since many substances have a marked buffer reaction.

The water-soluble "B" is not only soluble in water but can be dissolved in other reagents. Thus McCollum has shown that while benzene is of little value as an extractant of this vitamine, if we will first extract the vitamine with alcohol or water and deposit this on dextrin by evaporation it is then possible by shaking the activated dextrin with benzene to cause the vitamine to pass into solution in benzene. Voegtlin and Meyers have recently shown that it is soluble in olive oil and in oleic acid and their data suggest a new means of concentrating the substance which may be of value in tracing its character.

The "B" vitamine is relatively easily absorbed by finely divided precipitates. We have already referred to the use of fuller's earth for this purpose by Seidell. This adsorptive power sometimes manifests itself in the treatment of plant extracts. A watery extract of alfalfa can be made to throw down its protein complex by diluting it to 40 per cent with alcohol. Osborne reports however that this process frequently removes the vitamine also which appears to be thrown down with the precipitated material. This adsorptive power therefore often appears as a difficulty in the handling of the substance as well as a means of extraction. We have used Osborne's method with alfalfa extracts and find the above result is not by any means invariable, for in some of our extracts we retained the greater part of the vitamine. Kaolin and ordinary charcoal are not very good adsorbents but the latter can be activated to serve this purpose.

The elementary nature of the "B" vitamine remains a mystery. Extracts which contain it show the presence of nitrogen. Funk's earlier researches on yeast and rice polishings both yielded crystalline complexes which he analysed. His data on this subject follow:

A. The yeast complex

Crystals melting at 233. consisting of:

I. A complex melting at 229. and forming needles and prisms nearly insoluble in water and with the apparent formula of $C_{24}H_{19}O_2N_5$.

II. A complex melting at 222. and soluble in water. Formula $C_{29}H_{23}O_2N_5$.

III. Nicotinic acid melting at 235. $C_6H_5O_2N$.

B. The rice complex

Crystals melting at 233. consisting of:

I. A complex melting at 233. and with a formula of $C_{26}H_{20}O_9N_4$.

II. Nicotinic acid melting at 235. $C_6H_5O_2N$.

Funk held at the time that the possible nature of the compound was:

$$HN \mid \backslash OC \ C_{16}H_{18}O_6 \mid / HN$$

It was this idea that led him to call it an "amine."

We are unable at present to report any nearer approach to the elementary analysis and all attempts at purification have shown a tendency to make the active substance either disappear entirely or else distribute itself over the several fractions instead of concentrating itself in one. Its basic nature seems to be well established by its behavior with phosphotungstic acid and its ready adsorption by carbons activated to take up basic substances.

III. THE CHEMICAL PROPERTIES OF WATER-SOLUBLE "C"

The properties of this newest member of the family are still less defined. All are agreed that it is much more sensitive to heat and alkali than the other two. Temperatures above 50. are usually destructive though the time factor is extremely important as well as the reaction. Hess for example has found that the temperature used to pasteurize milk continued for some time, is more destructive to the vitamine than boiling water temperature continued for only a few minutes. The extent to which orange juice and tomato juice will resist high temperatures indicates the protective action of acids to be considerable.

Dr. Delf's experiments at the Lister Institute were especially directed to the behavior of this vitamine in cabbage. She first determined the minimum close of raw cabbage required to prevent scurvy in guinea pigs and found that it was less than 1.5 grams and more than 0.5 gram daily. When the cabbage was heated in water at 60. for an hour, symptoms of severe scurvy were just prevented by 5 grams of the cooked cabbage fed daily. By heating at 70? 80? 90?and 100?for the same length of time the 5 grams of cooked material could be made non-effective as a preventive. Her conclusions are that when cabbage is cooked for one hour at temperatures ranging from 80?to 100. the cabbage leaves lose about 90 per cent of the antiscorbutic power originally held by the raw equivalent. Sixty minutes at 60?or twenty minutes at 90?to 100?resulted in about 80 per cent destruction. Dr. Delf calls attention also to the fact that the effect of the heat is increased to only a slight degree by rise in temperature. Assuming that the effect of the rise is orderly, a temperature coefficient of 1.3 is indicated for each rise of 10. This low result suggests to Delf a contradiction to any theory which imputes to the vitamine enzyme or protein-like qualities and on the other hand suggests that the substance is much simpler in constitution. Her results also confirm Hoist and Frilich as showing its great sensitiveness at temperatures of 100?and below and obviously have a direct bearing upon cookery methods.

The substance is soluble in water and passes through a parchment membrane or a porcelain filter. Unlike the "B" it is apparently not adsorbed by fine precipitates such as fullers' earth or colloidal iron. Harden and Zilva showed that when a mixture of equal volumes of autolysed yeast and orange juice is treated with fuller's earth the "B" is removed and the "C" left unaltered. Eddy and La Mer have treated orange juice with fullers' earth and then tested the filtered off juice as cure and preventive of scurvy in guinea pigs. Their results showed that 6-2/3 cc. of the treated juice was curative, hence the loss due to adsorption must be less than 60 per cent to 70 per cent. Harden and Zilva were among the first to state that the vitamine is much more stable in acid than in alkali. They have shown, that even 1/50 N sodium hydrate at room temperature has a rapidly destructive effect. On the other hand Delf showed that when 0.5 gm. citric acid is added to the water in which germinated lentils are boiled, the loss of the antiscorbutic properties is, if anything, greater than when no addition of acid is made. She therefore concluded that in cooking vegetables there should be no addition of either acid or alkali to the cooking water if one wishes to conserve this vitamine. Sherman, La Mer, and Campbell have been engaged in experiments bearing on this point throughout the past two years. Some of their results have recently been published and their observations are worthy of special attention from their bearing on the character of reaction of the vitamine in general. They first proceeded to determine the amount of filtered tomato juice just necessary to produce scurvy in degrees extending from no protection to complete protection and they also constructed a basal diet which is apparently optimum in nutrients and all other factors except the "C" vitamine. They found that at the natural acidity of tomato juice (pH 4.2) boiling for one hour destroyed practically 50 per cent of the antiscorbutic power and by boiling for four hours they destroyed 70 per cent, which indicates that the curve of the destructive process tends to flatten more than that of a unimolecular reaction. This result was confirmed by heating experiments conducted at 60? 80?and 100? In all cases the temperature coefficients are low. (Q_10 equals 1.1-1.3) confirming Delf's results. When the natural acidity of the juice was first neutralized in whole or in part, the juice then boiled for an hour and immediately cooled and reacidified, it was found that at less than half neutralization (pH 5.1-4.9) the destructive effect of an hour's boiling was increased to 58 per cent. When alkali was added to an initial pH 11 (about N/40 titratable alkali to phenolphthalein) which fell to 9 during the hour's boiling the destructive effect was about 65 per cent. When reacidification was omitted and the neutralized boiled juice stored in a refrigerator for five days before using the destruction increased 90 to 95 per cent. These particular observations seem to confirm the view of Harden and Zilva that the vitamine is especially sensitive to alkali. Hess has recently reported that oxygen is destructive to this vitamine.

IV. PHYSIOLOGICAL PROPERTIES OF THE "A" VITAMINE

Most authorities are now agreed that both the "A" and "B" types are essential to growth. Rohmann still holds out against the vitamine hypothesis.

McCollum has recently pointed out that while rats do not have scurvy it does not at all follow that the absence of the "C" in their diet is immaterial, but that the contrary is true. Failure to grow, then, may manifest itself as a result of the absence of either of the first two types and possibly is affected by the absence of the "C." We have already seen how this failure may be utilized to measure the vitamine content of a source. The absence of the "A" type however may also manifest itself in another way, viz., by the development of an eye disease which McCollum first designated as xerophthalmia or dry eye and which the British authorities prefer to designate as keratomalacia. The failure of this result to always follow the absence of the "A" type in the diet has led some to question the specificity of this disease. While the infection of the eye is due to other agents the sum of the evidence supports McCollum and points to the absence of "A" as the true predisposing cause of the disease. Bulley, basing her claims on a study of some 500 rats fed on a synthetic diet, claims that the eye condition is not primarily due to a dietary deficiency but to an infection resulting from poor hygienic conditions. In reply to her contentions Emmett has reviewed his own data and presents them in the following summation:

RAT GROUPS	KIND OF VITAMINE ABSENT IN THE RATION	NUMBER CASES REPORTED	POSITIVE CASES OF XEROPH-THALMIA	PER CENT POSITIVE
A	Fat-soluble "A"	122	120	98
B	Water-soluble "B"	103	0	0
C	None	216	0	0

In these groups special hygienic measures were taken against infection. Furthermore repeated attempts were made to transmit the eye disease by using sterile threads, passing them carefully over the edges of the sore lids and then carefully inoculating the eyes of other rats. These attempts resulted negatively in all cases where the inoculated rats had plenty of the "A" vitamine. Treatment of advanced cases of sore eyes with a saturated solution of boric acid and also with a silver protein solution failed to relieve the condition while as little as 2 per cent of an extract containing the "A" vitamine when added to the ration, speedily resulted in cure and increase of weight. These results combined with similar data compiled by Osborne and Mendel seem to refute Bulley's contentions and to justify our acceptance of xeropthalmia as a specific vitamine deficiency disease.

Osborne and Mendel data Total No. No. with eye symptoms

Rats on diets deficient in A vitamine . . . . 136 69 " on diets " " B " . . . . 225 0 " on diets otherwise deficient . . . . 90 0 " on " experimental but probably adequate . 201 0 " on mixed food . . . . 348 0 _____ __

Totals 1000 69

On the other hand all workers know that rats often do develop and grow well for a considerable period of time on a diet free from the "A" and without manifesting the eye disease. The British authorities explain this by assuming that animals have the power to lay down a reserve of this vitamine on which they can draw in emergency. Sherman and his coworkers confirm this power to store the vitamine. Others have been led to explain their results as due to contamination of the basal diet. Daniels and Loughlin recently maintained that the commercial lard used in basal diets and assumed to be "A" vitamine-free was supplied with sufficient of the "A" to produce growth and prevent eye disease. Their views have failed of confirmation by Osborne and Mendel. It is evident therefore that these occasional lapses from specific response to absence of the "A" vitamine need further elucidation. It is equally manifest that in the majority of cases the absence of the "A" will result in both stunted growth and xeropthalmia. The appearance of the eye disease may be taken however, as a sure indication of the absence or deficiency in the "A" vitamine.

V. PHYSIOLOGICAL PROPERTIES OF THE "B" VITAMINE

Beri-beri is a disease that is described clinically as a form of severe peripheral neuritis and may appear in two well marked forms. In one type there is great wasting, anesthesia of the skin and finally paralysis of the limbs. In the other, the most marked symptom is excessive edema which may affect trunk, limbs and extremities. In severe cases the heart is usually involved and death may occur suddenly from heart failure.

Most observers assume that the antineuritic vitamine discovered by Funk and the water-soluble "B" are identical. This view is based on the fact that when sources which yield the water-soluble "B" in rat feeding are tested for antineuritic power these sources are apparently parallel in antineuritic power and growth production. Furthermore rats deprived of the water-soluble "B" develop polyneuroses identical in symptoms with those shown by rats and pigeons when the latter are placed on a polished rice diet. The British Medical Board has compiled the following table to support this view:

Table compiled from pages 35 and 86, British Medical Research Committee Report

THE FOODSTUFF	VALUE AS A SOURCE OF WATER-SOLUBLE "B" (SHOWN BY EXPERIMENTS WITH RATS)	VALUE AS A SOURCE OF ANTINEURETIC FACTOR OR ANTI-BERI-BERI FACTOR (SHOWN BY EXPERIMENTS WITH BIRDS)
Rice germ	+++	++++
Wheat germ	+++	+++
Yeast	+++	+++
Egg yolk	++	+++
Ox liver	++	+++
Wheat bran	+	++
Meat muscle	+	+
Milk	+++	Slight
Potatoes	+	+
Meat extract	0	0
White bread or flour	0	0
Polished rice	0	0

BEHAVIOR	WATER-SOLUBLE "B"	ANTINEURITIC VITAMINE
Solubility in water	Very soluble	Very soluble
Solubility in alcohol, dilute	Very soluble	Very soluble
Solubility in absolute alcohol	Insoluble	Insoluble
Solubility in ether, chloroform and benzene	Insoluble	Unusually insoluble but can be extracted with ether from fatty materials such as egg yolk
Stability to heat	Stable at 100 癈, destroyed rapidly at temperatures below 120?(in neutral or acid solution)	Destroyed very slowly at 10., more rapid at temperatures between 110 and 120.
Stability to drying	Stable	Stable
Stability to acids (hot dilute)	Moderately stable	Stable

Stability to acids | | (cold dilute) . . . | Stable | Stable Stability to alkalies | | (hot dilute) . . . | Rapidly destroyed | ? Stability to alkalies | | (cold dilute) . . . | Stable | In dialysis . . . . . | Passes through | Passes through | parchment membrane | parchment membrane In adsorption . . . . | Adsorbed from acid | Adsorbed from neutral | or neutral solution | solutions by fuller's | by fuller's earth, | earth, colloidal | charcoal, etc. | ferric hydroxide, | | animal charcoal,   etc.

_____|_____|_____
_____

Emmett has recently opposed this view and suggests that while the antineuritic factor and the growth factor are found in the same sources and have much in common it does not follow that they are identical and that his experiments tend to show that there are marked differences which suggest that the "B" type is not a single entity but a group. Mitchell has summarized very well the controversial phases of this question with an impartial review of the facts. One of strongest of the opposition arguments lies in the failure of milk to cure beri-beri except when administered in large quantities. This objection has been partly allayed by data bearing on the relation of the milk content to the food of the cow. Hess, Dutcher, Hart and Steenbock and others have adduced sufficient evidence to show that the vitamine content of the milk of a cow is largely determined by the cow's food and as a consequence the milk may be very poor in vitamine. It is obvious then that the failure of the milk to cure beri-beri in a given case might be due to this cause and not to lack of identity of the curative with the growth factor. Osborne and Mendel have also shown that milk in general must not be classed among the rich sources of the vitamine, even when the cow's food is rich in vitamine. The principal facts in the controversy have been presented and at present the evidence for regarding the vitamines identical seems to be preponderant.

Recently Auguste Lumiere in Paris has put forth the view that polyneuritis is not merely a vitamine deficiency disease but a nutriment deficiency disease. He reports that he fed birds on a starvation diet, but with plenty of vitamine "B". These birds developed polyneuritis and were cured by adding to the diet plenty of polished rice. The view he wishes us to take is that all factors must be present and that the absence of the nutriment is as important as the absence of the vitamine.

In the field of nutrition the absence of the "B" type is particularly marked by the behavior of the deprived animal. Rats transferred from a vitamine-free diet to one containing the "B" only, make a much more rapid recovery toward normal (even in the absence of the "A") than do animals transferred from the vitamine-free diet to one containing the "A" and not the "B". This initial jump from addition of the "B" will not continue long in the absence of the "A", as a general rule. Hess believes that in some of his infants he was able to show markedly successful growth on the diet deficient in the "A" but rich in the "B". It is not certain however that his diets were sufficiently devoid of the "A" factor to be declared "A" vitamine-free and we know little of the amount of the "A" necessary to normal infant growth. All results however show that both "A" and "B" are necessary to growth production and though the term growth vitamine was applied to the "A" originally the distinction is one that should be rejected, for both "A" and "B" and possibly "C" are all entitled to this name.

The manner in which the "B" vitamine acts is still obscure. Voegtlin some time ago tried to demonstrate that it was identical with secretin and stimulated pancreatic flow. Recent work at the Johns Hopkins University by Cowgill and by Aurep and Drummond in England has failed to confirm this. One of its most marked immediate effects is increase in appetite. Karr in Mendel's laboratory has shown that dogs which refused their basal diet would resume eating it if they were allowed to ingest separately a little dried yeast. Karr studied the metabolism of these dogs as regards nitrogen partition but the results give little data that is explicatory of the behavior of the vitamine. In 1915 the author was able to bring about marked immediate improvement and the ultimate recovery of a number of infants who were of the marasmic type by merely increasing the "B" vitamine content of their food. In these cases the vitamine was carried by Lloyd's reagent and administered mixed with cereal, or the crude extract was combined with the milk. The pancreas of the sheep was the source used. In these cases the growth curve changed abruptly from a decline to a sharp rise and this increase in weight continued and was accompanied by all the other signs of improved nutrition including increase in appetite. The change in the growth curve from decline to rise was accomplished without increasing or changing the basal diet but as the appetite increased the food had naturally to be increased to keep pace. In these cases the effect of the vitamine was to enable the child to utilize its normal food and to increase its appetite for it. This action certainly suggests stimulation of digestive glands. It also showed that even though the diet may contain the vitamine as was the case in the milk fed to these children the addition of the vitamine in concentrated form often gives an upward push that the food mixture fails to accomplish. Daniels and Byfield have recently confirmed the effect of increased "B" in infant growth. Cramer has suggested in a paper published recently in The American Journal of Physiology that the fatty tissue about the suprarenals may be a depository of vitamine and that in the absence of vitamine this tissue loses its supply and that this is the explanation of lessened activity of that gland in certain metabolic disturbances. This idea tends to support the idea that vitamines are gland stimulants or hormones and the word food hormone has been suggested to describe them on that account. A few years ago Calkins and Eddy tried to determine the effect of the vitamine on the single cell by use of the paramecium but the results of the experiments failed to show a vitamine requirement on the part of these animals. McDougall has recently suggested that the vitamines produce their effect on yeast cells by increasing hydration. Unfortunately nearly all stimuli which produce growth are accompanied by hydration effects and it is difficult to feel that this is a specific vitamine effect although without denying the possibility. Dutcher has tried to show that vitamines have a relation to oxidation effects. He observed that the issues of polyneuritic birds showed a marked reduction in catalase and that this catalase was restorable by curing the birds with vitamine. The main difficulty lies in the conflexity of factors that function between cause and effect.

_1_. On the twentieth day the patient developed a cough. _2_. On the twenty-first day the cereal was reduced from three times a day to twice a day. The patient cried during the night. _3_. On the twenty- second day the stools showed free starch. _4_. On the twenty-third day an anal abscess was opened. The stools continued to show free starch until the twenty-fifth day. _5_. On the twenty-fifth day the stools showed soluble starch but no free starch. _6_. On the twenty-seventh day the appetite was good and there was no starch. _7_. From the twenty-eighth to the forty-third day no starch was observed in the stools. _8_. On the thirty-first day the patient developed a cough. _9_. From the forty-ninth day to the time of discharge three tablespoonsful of orange juice were given daily. _10_. On the seventy-third day the patient developed a bronchitis and mustard paste was applied every four hours up to the eighty-fourth day.

_V1_ = From the twenty-first day to the forty-third day the patient received each day 2 grams of Lloyd powder, activated with pancreatic vitamin. The powder was administered by mixing 1 gram. with each cereal feeding. The result was 20 ounces gain in twenty-two days, a normal growth.

_V2_ = After a period of ten days without vitamin, during which the patient settled down to a level growth curve, the treatment described under V1 was resumed. This was continued from the fifty-third to the seventy-sixth day. The result was the resumption of growth but at a slower rate; 8 ounces were gained in twenty-three days. During the latter part of the period the patient developed a bronchitis. At the end of this period the patient was placed on a whole milk formula. From that time to the time of discharge the patient grew normally.--From the _American Journal of Diseases of Children,_ 1917, xiv, 189.]

These views are at best speculations. The literature is singularly lacking in detailed metabolic analyses of excreta of animals during vitamine stimulation and we know nothing of the possibilities of overdosage, for in all the work done it has been generally assumed that the presence of an amount greater than that necessary to produce normal growth is not material.

The exact manner of the vitamine's action then remains to be determined and it is obvious that this solution will come much more rapidly if we can first identify the substance chemically.

VI. THE PHYSIOLOGICAL PROPERTIES OF THE "C" VITAMINE

The steps that led to the acceptance of scurvy as a vitamine deficiency disease have already been discussed and show how the vitamine acts in such a disease. Practically all the work done with this vitamine to date has been concerned either with dosage or with reaction to heat, drying, etc. The only paper that we have seen that suggests another function than antiscorbutic power for this vitamine is the one by McCollum and Parsons in which they suggest that even in animals where scurvy does not exist, the presence of this factor may be necessary to normal metabolism. The following table gives some of the data compiled by the British workers as to the antiscorbutic

Table compiled from, page 44, British Medical Research Committee Report

FOODSTUFF	VALUE AGAINST SCURVY	MINIMUM DAILY RATION NECESSARY TO PREVENT SCURVY IN GUINEA PIGS
Cereals:		
Whole grains	0	Germ . . . .
Bran	0	Endosperm 0
Pulses:		
Whole dry	0	
Germinated (lentils)	++	5.0 grams
Vegetables:		
Cabbage (raw)	++++	1.0 gram
Cabbage (cooked one-half hour at 100)	++	5.0 grams
Runner beans (green pods)	+++	5.0 grams
Carrot (juice)	+	20.0 cc.
Beet root (juice)	+	More than 20 cc.
Swede (juice)	+++	2.5 cc.
Potatoes (cooked one-half hour at 100)	+	20.0 grams
Onions	+	
Desiccated vegetables	0 to +	60.0 grams expressed as equivalent in fresh cabbage
Fruits:		
Lemon juice (fresh)	++++	1.5 cc.
Lemon juice (preserved)	++	5.0 cc.
Orange juice (fresh)	++++	1.5 cc.
Lime juice (fresh)	++	10.0 cc.
Lime juice (preserved)	0 to +	
Grapes	Less than +	More than 20.0 grams
Apples	Less than +	
Apples dried	Less than +	
Tamarind dried	Less than +	
Mango	Less than +	
Kokum	Less than +	
Meat:		
Raw, juice	Less than +	More than 20 cc.
Tinned	0	

A glance at this table shows the richest sources (see also table on page 59.) To these must be added canned tomato juice which Hess has shown practically equal to orange juice in efficiency and uses with infants in the same quantity. This discovery is of great value in instances where the cost of orange juice is often prohibitive.

La Mer and Campbell have presented some evidence to show that the antiscorbutic vitamine has a direct effect upon the adrenal glands. In their scurvy cases they find definite evidence of the enlargement or hypertrophy of this organ. Whether it affects other organs or not it remains to be shown.

CHAPTER VII

HOW TO UTILIZE THE VITAMINE IN DIETS

In the preceding chapters it has been the aim to present the findings of the principal workers in the field. In attempting to summarize the work of so widely scattered a group as are now engaged in vitamine research it is impossible to cover completely the many investigations and it is inevitable that some work will have been overlooked, but the foregoing covers at least the principal data on the subject. What is the bearing of all this information on human behavior and what lessons can the layman draw from it that is of direct application to him? Let us first consider this question from the dietary viewpoint.

I. INFANT NUTRITION

The limited character of the infant's diet has made the consideration of vitamine content in his diet much more important than in the case of the adult with the latter's wide variety of choice. It is evident from the previous data that a growing infant must not only be provided with a sufficient supply of calories, nutrients and salts, but must also have a liberal supply of the three vitamines. Milk has in general been classed as adequate in all these features, but the vitamine researches have forced us to reconsider our views in regard to this staple.

The first point to be borne in mind is that the vitamine content of either cow or human milk is dependent primarily upon the food eaten by the producer of the milk. In other words milk is merely a mobilization of the vitamines eaten and if the diet is to yield vitamine-rich milk it must itself be rich in these factors. Many a cow produces milk low in vitamine content and the same is true of nursing mothers. There are many "old wives" prejudices in regard to what food a lactating mother may eat and unfortunately many of these prejudices are extremely injurious and false. One of them is the prejudice against green vegetables. Experience has shown that under ordinary conditions such vegetables are well tolerated by the mother and from their content of vitamine it is evident that they are suppliers of these factors. In the case of the cow the fact that cereals are poor in some of the vitamines and green grasses rich therein, teaches a lesson that bears directly upon winter feeding of cattle if the milk supply is to be used for infants. We need a series of diets and cattle foods for just this purpose of insuring the proper vitamine content in milk. The preceding tables will enable one to develop such diets fairly satisfactorily, but more data is urgently needed.

The second point in regard to milk lies in the effect of pasteurization. This measure is now well nigh universal and in America at least has played a tremendous part in the reduction of infant mortality, especially during the summer months. At present, however, we know that this treatment while removing dangerous germs may also eliminate the antiscorbutic factor. The sensible attitude then is to recognize this fact and if a clean whole milk is not available retain the pasteurization and meet the vitamine deficiency by other agents. Such agents are orange juice and tomato juice and experience has already shown that these juices can be well tolerated by infants much earlier than used to be thought possible.

While the pasteurization does not appreciably affect the content of "A" or "B" vitamines, the variability in content of these vitamines in milk indicates that it may at times be necessary to supplement them in the diet. In this connection it must be borne in mind that cereals vary widely in content and cannot be, as they often are now, considered equivalent in growth stimulation power. This is a subject that needs special attention on the part of vitamine experts and dietitians and finally by the food manufacturers. A good vitamine-rich cereal combination would form an excellent adjuvant to infant dietaries after they reach the age of tolerance to such a diet. But even before that time the expressed juice of various vegetables as well as fruits is found to be well tolerated when mixed with the milk or given separately, and carrot and spinach juice are now being used in this connection with good results. These juices like orange juice contain the B type in abundance and there is no doubt that in their stimulation to the appetite they play an important part in making the desirable daily gain.

Fortunately for the layman he has in the scales a good indicator of the normal progress of his child and so long as growth is normal he can fairly assume that the diet is adequate but if the scales say otherwise it is time for him to seek advice and then he is wise who insures that his medical adviser knows the newer aspects of nutrition. The parent can do this only by proper selection, but with a little knowledge he can soon satisfy himself as to whether his pediatrist is the right sort and it is one of the purposes of this text to bring home to the layman his responsibility in this matter.

There has grown up in this country a great regard for prepared milk substitutes in infant feeding and a wide usage of condensed milks, reinforced milks, diluted milk formulae, etc. All such preparations must be examined anew in the light of the vitamine discoveries and unless the given preparation can show a clean bill of health in vitamine content, it should be either discarded or properly supplemented.

As children grow up, it is fortunate that in their wider choice of dietaries the danger of vitamine deficiency decreases. But even in childhood it is unsafe to rely too much on chance. In this country there are well deserving movements on foot to attract the parents of the community to the necessity of attention to simple standards of growth progress, and clinics for this purpose are appearing in increasing numbers with each year. Such movements are to be most heartily approved. It is also possible in these measures to not only build better children, but to make the children themselves intelligent in their rejection of unsuitable combinations and in that way not only conserve their own health, but provide an educated body of citizens to pass on the knowledge to future generations. In a school in New York City I recently had occasion to discuss the school lunch room and its offerings with the children of the school in the light of vitamine discoveries. The keenness and intelligence shown by the children in the discussion that followed has convinced me that in this matter of vitamines the children themselves can be relied upon to assist materially in the matter of better food combinations and intelligent selection.

Finally it must be noted that one of the most common of infant deficiencies is the failure of the bones to lay down lime. The effect of this failure is commonly described as rickets. The British workers consider that this deficiency is a lack of vitamine "A." Their views have been set forth at greatest length by Mellanby, the principal worker in this subject. While this view is still debatable and in this country it is not yet accepted, one fact has come out in the controversy and that is the remarkable value of cod-liver oil as a preventive of rickets. It may be that the power of the oil is due to its "A" vitamine content in which it is known to be rich, or it may be due to a new vitamine, but the fact that the oil is a preventive in this respect gives the pediatrist another agent to insure normal growth. The various views on the causes of rickets are set forth more in detail in

Chapter VIII.

II. ADULT DIETS

A study of the dietary habits of various sections of the United States shows that there is a very general tendency on the part of the majority of the people to confine their foods to a meat, potato, and cereal diet. The use of salads is looked upon by many sections as a foreign affectation and too little attention is paid to the value of eggs, milk and cheese. Enough has been said already to show that these latter articles have much more than an esthetic value and one of the missions of the nutrition expert must be to show the people why dairy products and salads must become features in the every-day meals of the every-day people. And even if the salads are still unappreciated, it is necessary that cooked green vegetables occupy more of a position in the menu than is too often the case.

There has recently appeared a crusade for the eating of yeast cakes. The claim made for their use rests on a perfectly firm basis, they are rich in the "B" vitamine, the proteins of the yeast cake are of good quality and the cake contains no ingredients poisonous to man. Many people are reporting beneficial effects from their use. Is there any lesson to be drawn from this experiment? I feel that the very fact that benefits have resulted from this yeast feeding is excellent evidence of lack of the vitamine in the diets of the people affected and a clear argument that the dietary habits of many people need adjustment to a higher vitamine content. Whether it is necessary to use yeast cakes or any other concentrate of vitamine, depends entirely upon whether the ordinary diet is lacking in these factors and my first advice in the matter would be to make if possible a selection of the vitamine containing foods and see if normal conditions did not result before utilizing foods whose taste is not pleasing or which are taken as medicine. For it is an old experience that medicines will be taken only so long as the patient is sick and perhaps it is just as well so. In other words I believe it is possible with intelligent selection based on such tables as are given in

Chapter IV

for people to secure from the butcher and the grocer all their requirements of these vitamines as a part of their regular palatable diet. To those who have neglected this selection and find remedy in concentrates, that fact should lead them to reconstruct their diet rather than persist in dependence on the medicine to correct faulty diet. In other words the same arguments apply to the use of medicinal concentrates of vitamines as applies to the use of laxatives. At times these substances are very valuable as cures, but it is better by far to so regulate the dietary habits as to avoid the necessity for their use.

Another phase of this matter that promises to develop in the near future as a result of the vitamine hypothesis is a reform in food manufacture. There has been a strong tendency during the past two decades to "purify" food products. The genesis of this tendency is to be found in a highly laudable ambition to force the manufacturer to eliminate impurities and adulterations and provide clean, wholesome, sanitary food. Unfortunately in attempting to meet this demand on the part of the public, the food manufacturer has sometimes neglected to seek advice from the nutrition expert and the latter has failed to appreciate the need of advice. The net result has been to discover that Nature is often a better chemist than man and has a much better knowledge of what man needs in his diet than the chemist. The chemist employed by the manufacturer has, as a result, gone to such a limit in his development of purification methods as to often eliminate the essential nutrients and the result has been foods that will stand analysis for pure nutrients, but which will not stand Nature's analysis for dietary efficiency. As a secondary result of this tendency we have acquired habits that in many cases must either be broken or must have grafted on to them other habits which shall remedy the defective ones. Take the milling of wheat as an example. Nature put into the wheat grain most of the elements needed by man and in the early days he was content to grind up the whole grain and find it palatable. The craze for purity as expressed by color has gradually replaced this whole meal wheat with a beautiful white product that is largely pure starch with a few of the proteins retained. And the principal protein retained lacks one of the greatest essentials for growth while the vitamines have all been practically eliminated with the grain germ. Intelligence tells us then that if, having formed the habit, we will persist in our appetite for white flour we must see to it that the protein deficiency of the latter and its lack of vitamines is compensated for by supplementing the diet with the food-stuffs in which these are rich. We may in other words retain our bad habits in taste if we will graft on to them the attention to the eliminated factors and their substitution in other form.

In general then, the adult needs to review his feeding habits and analyze them in the light of our new knowledge. For this purpose the tables of

Chapter IV

supply data useful so far as vitamines are concerned, but it will be perhaps worth while to repeat here some of this data in more generalized form.

a. Sources of the "A" vitamine

Its most abundant sources are milk, butter, egg yolk fat, and the green leaves of plants usually classed as salads. Cabbage, lettuce, spinach and carrots contain this substance in considerable quantity. The germ of cereals is fairly rich in the factor, but the rest of the grain is deficient and white flours are therefore poorer than whole meals in this respect. Cooking temperatures have little effect on this vitamine and hence little attention need be paid to cooking temperatures as far as this vitamine is concerned.

b. Sources of the "B" vitamine

Its principal sources outside of yeast are the seeds of plants and the eggs and milk of animals. Meat contains relatively little of this substance but glandular organs such as the liver and pancreas are fairly rich in it. In the seeds the distribution is general throughout the whole body of the seed in the case of beans, peas, etc., but in the cereal grains it is largely restricted to the embryo portion and hence a high degree of milling tends to reduce the per cent of this factor in any highly milled cereal. White flour and polished rice are notable examples of deficiency of "B" vitamine due to this milling process. Fruits such as oranges, tomatoes, and lemons are good sources and there is a fair amount present in the apples and grapes and other common food fruits. Many vegetables show it in fair abundance, notably potatoes, carrots, and turnips, but the rule is not general for beets are extremely poor in this factor. Nuts are also good sources. Eggs, milk and cheese contain it in fair abundance. Cooking temperatures have little effect on this type if the temperature does not climb above the boiling point and if the cooking water is not "alkaline." In the latter case it becomes necessary to determine the extent of destruction and either eat enough to insure protection, or reform the method of cookery.

c. Sources of the "C" vitamine

Its richest sources are vegetables such as cabbage, swedes, turnips, lettuce and watercress; fruits such as lemons, oranges, raspberries and tomatoes. Certain of the vegetables such as potatoes have a substantial value in this respect, but meat and most prepared milks are low in antiscorbutic values. The susceptibility of this vitamine to drying, heat and alkali, make it necessary to scrutinize your cooking methods very carefully in order not to ruin a good source by a poor preparation of it for the table.

CHAPTER VIII

AVITAMINOSES OR THE DISEASES THAT RESULT FROM VITAMINE DEFICIENCIES

A survey of the vitamines would be incomplete without a discussion of the vitamine deficiency diseases in particular, though many of the facts already cited obviously bear on the treatment and prevention of such diseases.

The idea of "avitaminoses" or vitamine deficiency as the cause of a disease of a specific nature was set forth in detail by Funk in his book Die Vitamine. In his discussion of this view he suggests several types that would, he felt, on examination prove to be due to the absence of a vitamine in the diet. Of these predicted types beri-beri was the only one to be established in 1913. Scurvy has now been added to the fold and rickets or rachitis seems well on the way to acceptance though the specific vitamine absent in this case is not yet positively identified. Pellagra still resists the efforts of the vitamine hypothesis to bend it to that theory and its etiology is still obscure.

I. BERI-BERI

This disease while specifically confined to the oriental in the mind of the student can be justly considered of much wider distribution for the mild forms of malnutrition associated with a deficiency in the "B" vitamine are less acute manifestations of this disease. The disease is not likely to become marked in well nourished districts in its acute form, but in famine districts its incidence is always possible. It would be more than possible were it not for the fact that famine tends to eliminate the highly milled cereals and throw the people back on to the whole grain, peas and beans, which are rich in the preventive factor. But when for any reason diets become limited extra attention is demanded in regard to their selection and preparation. The main characteristics of this disease have already been fully covered in what precedes and need not be repeated here.

II. SCURVY

This disease, like beri-beri has already been fully discussed in what precedes. One of the striking discoveries of this subject has been the retreat from favor of the time-honored lime juice which is now found to be much less potent than oranges, lemons, or even canned tomato juice and which on preservation loses practically all its potency. In the modern hospital, cases of scurvy rarely appear outside of occasional infant cases and it might appear that the problem of scurvy prevention is peculiarly that of the sailor, the explorer and the army rationer. Nevertheless an insufficient supply of the "C" vitamine may retard growth and well being in the individual without manifesting itself in its more acute form of scurvy. In a recent review Hess states: "It is hardly an exaggeration to state that in the temperate zones the development or non-development of scurvy depends largely on the potato crop." "This is attributed in part to the fact that the potato is an excellent antiscorbutic, but to a greater extent because it is consumed during the winter in amounts that exceed the combined total of all other vegetables." To the public and to the food purveyor there is a definite problem in how to best supply the preventive and how best to concentrate and preserve the sources of this vitamine without injury to its potency. The following observation is therefore appended as bearing on this point. In the absence of fruits or other high potency sources it is possible to develop this factor in cereal grains by the simple expediency of sprouting. If seeds are soaked in water for twenty-four hours and then kept moist for from one to three days with the free access of air, sprouts will develop whose content of the antiscorbutic vitamine is comparable to that of many fresh vegetables, even though the dry seeds themselves have little of this factor. In other words the germination process is a synthesiser of the vitamine. This observation may be of value where fruits and vegetables are scarce or expensive. On account of cooking effects, it cannot be too often reiterated that raw fruits, vegetables and salads, are of more value than cooked forms of these same sources and that drying processes are extremely destructive where heat enters into the drying process. Vacuum drying seems to be much less destructive and it may be possible to develop the drying of vegetables to a point where retention of this vitamine factor is practical. At present all dried vegetables should be regarded with suspicion as a source of vitamine "C." Expressed juices may often be used where the whole vegetable is scarce or incompatible and this fact is one to be borne in mind by the worker in famine districts.

III. RACHITIS (RICKETS)

This disease is engaging the attention of many workers on both sides of the Atlantic at the present time. In England the principal contributor is Dr. Mellanby, who has accumulated evidence which he believes indicates that the preventive factor is the A vitamine. This view is not yet accepted as conclusive by the American workers. McCollum, Howland, Park, and others at Johns Hopkins University have experimented with various rickets-producing diets and while the principal deficiency in these diets seems to be Ca salts and the A vitamine they do not consider that the disease can as yet be traced to deficiency in any one factor. Hess has called attention to several new features and the significance of some older measures. He has shown on the one hand that cod-liver oil is almost a specific remedy for the disease but that this remedy is not replaceable by other rich sources of the A vitamine. He has also recently shown that hygienic measures may have an influence. Schmorl showed that the disease was seasonal, a high rate maintaining in the winter months and a lower rate in the summer months. Hess has recently reported beneficial results from use of the ultra-violet rays which he uses as a substitute for sunlight. The results seem to confirm Schmorl's view that the sunlight of the summer months is a preventive factor. He has also suggested that the specific effect of the cod-liver oil might be due to a new vitamine, Vitamine D? On the other hand Zilva and Miura in England have recently shown that crude cod-liver oil is something like two hundred and fifty times as rich in vitamine A as butter fat, which tends to support the British view that the A vitamine is the antirachitic factor.

Sherman and Pappenheimer have recently shown that the phosphates exert a marked preventive effect on rickets and suggest that the utilization of the calcium by the individual may be determined in part by this factor.

The views in brief are now in an extremely chaotic state and it is impossible at present to determine whether rickets is a true avitaminose or a consequence of deficiency in a series of factors. It is however certain that the disease in its subacute forms is extremely wide-spread among infants and that its prevention can be most easily secured by the addition of cod-liver oil to the diet. In this procedure warning is necessary that the cod-liver oil be as pure a product of oil as possible, since the market preparations are often almost devoid of the true oil and hence of the curative agent.

IV. PELLAGRA

This disease has been the subject of exhaustive inquiry and study on this side of the Atlantic and the findings of the various investigating boards have added much to the prevention and cure of the scourge, but have failed as yet to agree on any one etiological factor. The best recent review of the current findings is to be found in an article by Voegtlin published as Reprint 597 of the Public Health Reports of the United States Public Health Service. His conclusions may be quoted in full as representing the latest summary of evidence now extant:

1. The hypothesis that there is a causal relation between pellagra and a restricted vegetable diet has been substantiated by direct proof to this effect and has led to results of considerable practical and scientific value.

2. The metabolism in pellagra shows certain definite changes from the normal, which point to decreased gastric secretion and increased intestinal putrefaction.

3. In the treatment and prevention of pellagra, diet is the essential factor. The disease can be prevented by an appropriate change in diet without changing other sanitary conditions.

4. A diet of the composition used by pellagrins prior to their attack by the disease leads to malnutrition and certain pathological changes in animals, resembling those found in pellagra. A typical pellagrous dermatitis has not been observed in animals. Pellagrous symptoms have been produced in man by the continued consumption of a restricted vegetable diet.

5. The nature of the dietary effect has not been discovered, although certain observations point to a combined deficiency in some of the recognized dietary factors as the cause of the pellagrous syndrome.

In elaborating on conclusion 5 Voegtlin states that:

The conception that pellagra is due to a dietary deficiency is, therefore, not contradicted by the available evidence. This does not imply that the disease is necessarily due to a deficiency of diet in a specific substance such as the hypothetical pellagra vitamine of Funk (1913). It is much more likely that the pellagrous syndrome is caused by a combination of the deficiencies in some of the well recognized food factors.

V. OTHER AVITAMINOSES

The role of the vitamine in the nutrition and growth of organisms other than the man is becoming a matter of interest in various ways. The construction of culture media for various strains of bacteria and the conditions favorable or unfavorable to their growth, are features of study in which the new hypothesis has demanded attention. It has already been claimed that vitamines are essential to the growth of the meningococcus, the influenza bacillus, the typhoid bacillus, the gonococcus, the pneumococcus Type I, Streptococcus hemolyticus, the diptheria bacillus, the Bacillus pertussis and certain soil organisms. If these views are confirmed it becomes evident that the means for prevention of the development of these forms may lie in the control of the vitamine content of the materials on which these forms thrive and that in the study of these types it may be possible to speed up the incubation of strains and thus hasten diagnostic measures by introducing the necessary vitamines into the culture media. These observations merely suggest the possible widening of the scope of the vitamine study in the service of man and give added reason for our keeping pace with the strides made in this particular field.

###